What Seems To Be The Problem?

What Seems To Be The Problem?

A doctor's story about courage, compasion, and a new way to care

Dr Laura Marshall-Andrews

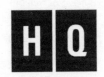

ONE PLACE. MANY STORIES

AUTHOR'S NOTE
Some names and events have been changed to protect the privacy of the individuals involved.

HQ
An imprint of HarperCollins*Publishers* Ltd
1 London Bridge Street
London SE1 9GF

www.harpercollins.co.uk

HarperCollins*Publishers*
1st Floor, Watermarque Building, Ringsend Road
Dublin 4, Ireland

This edition 2022

1

First published in Great Britain by
HQ, an imprint of HarperCollins*Publishers* Ltd 2022

ISBN: 978-0-00-844502-7

MIX
Paper from
responsible sources
FSC
www.fsc.org   FSC™ C007454

This book is produced from independently certified FSC™ paper
to ensure responsible forest management.

For more information visit: www.harpercollins.co.uk/green

This book is set in 11.7/16 pt Minion by Type-it AS, Norway

Printed and Bound in the UK using 100% Renewable Electricity at
CPI Group (UK) Ltd, Croydon, CR0 4YY

For Will, Josh, Danny, and Tassia,
who make everything worthwhile.

Contents

Introduction   1

PART 1: BEGINNING OUR JOURNEY   5

   1: Dreams   7

   2: Here comes Big Pharma   51

   3: N=1   60

   4: Quality   66

PART 2: CARING   79

   5: Fragmentation   81

   6: Pain   96

   7: Ethics   119

   8: Power   139

PART 3: FIGHTING FOR SURVIVAL   149

   9: Error   151

   10: Trial   181

   11: Death and life   187

PART 4: PANDEMIC   203

    12: Warnings   205

    13: Strength   215

    14: Lockdowns   229

    15: Hope   246

Epilogue   256

Acknowledgements   258

'If you have the choice between being kind or being clever, choose kind.'

R.J. PALACIO, *Wonder*

'Society today is being fragmented by a way of thinking that is inherently short-sighted because it disregards the full horizon of truth ... It ignores the very principles that enable us to live and flourish in unity, order and harmony.'

POPE BENEDICT XVI

Introduction

My surgery finished late on the day I was strangled.

My patient, Sarah, had about her the air of a recent escapee. I had treated her before and knew her mental health could be very up and down. But that day she looked particularly disconcerting. Her dark black hair was untamed, and her skin sallow with large dark circles around her wild eyes. She rushed into my consulting room followed by a man I recognised as another mental health patient of ours.

'I feel wild, I feel crazy.' Sarah was writhing as she spoke, pulling at her neck and the top of her shirt.

'She does,' the man behind her said to me over her shoulder, nodding vigorously.

They had met at a mental health day event at the surgery, he explained. He looked to be in a state of panic. This was not uncommon for him as he lived his life in a fairly constant state of panic, but there was a different urgency about him that day.

'She's been trying to attack people on the way here,' he said. 'She even tried to attack an old lady.'

Sarah nodded in agreement, widening her eyes and throwing her head back.

'Okay, well, just take a seat.' I gestured to the chair by my desk.

My consulting room was in the shape of a small reversed L, with the desk tucked into the short arm of the L to maximise space for the patient and the couch. It was an arrangement I was starting to regret as I suddenly felt very cornered.

'I can't sit down! I'm wild. I feel dangerous. I need to be admitted!' Her voice increased in energy and volume as she spoke.

'Okay, Sarah, I will just call Millview,' I said, moving my hand slowly to the phone and picking up the receiver. Millview is our local psychiatric hospital. It is not a pleasant place. Most of its patients spend their time trying to escape, and so wanting to be admitted there was in itself pretty indicative of a delusional state of mind.

I kept my eyes on Sarah as I dialled the number.

The ward clerk answered and put Graham, the team leader, on the line.

I explained the situation.

'Oh yes – I know Sarah,' he said, too quickly. 'I absolutely don't think admission is the right thing for her. I think she is best off in the community.'

'She says she is going to attack someone.'

'Well, yes – she does attack people. She's attacked me.' He paused as if this was somehow reassuring. I supposed that the fact that he was still alive was positive. That said, one couldn't tell down the phone whether or not he had suffered some sort of disfiguring disablement.

'Okay, so what should I do?'

'Call her community team. They might be able to help her.'

'Right,' I said. I certainly didn't feel right, but then I wasn't really in the sort of situation where I was expecting to.

Calling the community team is never straightforward. It is hopelessly understaffed, and it's almost impossible to get through to anyone. I ended up leaving three or four messages on different voicemails.

I turned back to Sarah. 'I'm trying to get you seen at home,' I explained.

'I can't go home – I'm going to kill someone!' she shouted. 'I need to be admitted! I feel dangerous!' And with that, she launched herself at me and grabbed my neck.

Time seemed to slow down as we pivoted backwards and forwards in a strange dance. Sarah was trying to strangle me, and I was trying to push her off. I had the palm of my right hand placed against her forehead, pushing it back. Her mouth was wide open and her chin extended towards me. Behind her, her friend was flapping his arms up and down shouting, 'Don't kill the doctor!' I could feel Sarah's thumb on my larynx and the blood backing up into my head. Fortunately I have long Neanderthal-type arms and I was able to stretch her forehead back so much that her grip on my neck loosened.

Spotting an opportunity, I managed to wrestle her to the ground and place a knee on her chest, which kept her still for long enough for me to grab the phone and dial 999.

We stayed on the ground for what seemed like an eternity. Every so often, Sarah would thrash around under my knee, but my full weight was on her and I had her arms pinned to the ground on either side. The police arrived quickly – two officers with walkie-talkies buzzing at their shoulders – and with them came a sense of safety. As soon as they walked into the room, I burst into tears.

I was trying to explain what had happened when Sarah launched herself at me again, and the police jumped into action. They held her arms behind her and turned her round so she was bent over and pressed into the examination couch with her head turned to one side.

'Okay, doc, we'll take it from here. Does she take any calming medication or anything?'

'Give me some diazepam!' Sarah shouted from her compromised position. The couch roll (a long strip of thin, changeable paper that covers the couch) was getting caught in her mouth. She tried to move it with her tongue. Saliva dribbled onto the tissue, which clung to her bottom lip. I put out my hand to help clean it off, but thought better of it as she growled at me.

Diazepam is an addictive sedative medication. I am usually very careful about using it, but this did seem like the perfect opportunity. 'Hold on,' I said, and rushed next door to my practice nurse.

I started shaking as the adrenalin hit me. 'Fi, I need some diaz- epam,' I said. 'Sarah has just tried to strangle me.' My voice rose in pitch at the end.

Fiona got up quickly and went to the locked drugs cabinet.

'Sit down, dear,' she said as she gave me two large tablets in a little plastic pot. 'Take these,' she said, and patted my shoulder as she handed me the glass of water she had filled at the sink.

'Not for me! For Sarah!'

I went back into the consulting room and gave Sarah the medica- tion. The police escorted her away and drove her to Millview.

I took a deep breath and called my next patient. She had been sitting resignedly outside my door, waiting for the screaming and shouting and police intervention to be over.

She came in and sat down. Our consultation began, with both of us pretending that everything was fine. It definitely wasn't. Underneath the desk, my hands were still shaking. My concern for Sarah fought with the basic response of anyone who is physically attacked – fear and shock. Just behind that was my deep exasperation with a healthcare system that was letting her down so badly.

Working as a doctor gives me deep joy and pride – but, let's be honest, there are times it scares the hell out of me.

PART 1

Beginning our journey

CHAPTER 1

Dreams

In the early 2000s, I was working as a GP in a practice in Brighton, Sussex. It was quite small, and run by just two of us, me and another GP, Jonathan. Jonathan was fun. He was a larger-than-life character, and I liked him. He had large frizzy hair and large features in his large face. We worked well together, but I found him rather old school. He held the views he held, and what he said went.

Still, I loved my patients, and knew how lucky I was that my work gave me real satisfaction. It also allowed me to balance my professional life with my family – my husband and our three kids, who were still quite young back then. I recognised how fortunate I was to have this sense of balance, considering how hard it is for so many people to find. We had a routine that worked for us all.

I'd always wanted to be a doctor. After years of rigorous studying, my peers and I had been spewed out of med school with the values and opinions of our time. We worshipped the gods of mass trial data and clinical evidence. We knew that our scientific knowledge was king.

And then, so slowly that I hardly noticed it at first, my ideas about medicine began to shift and change. I observed more and more instances where patients responded unexpectedly to treatments. I would start them on a medication that, according to the textbooks and literature, was supposed to take two weeks to offer any improvement in symptoms. It was baffling to me that a good percentage of people would come back immediately better and some would show no improvement for weeks and weeks, if at all.

People, I realised, are not textbooks. They are much more complicated than that – and far more interesting. Maybe, I thought, we don't know everything about what causes illness and wellness. Maybe things are happening in medicine that we don't yet fully understand.

I didn't say anything to Jonathan about what was running through my mind. I suspected that he wouldn't agree with me about any of it. But what, I started to wonder, was really going on?

*

I met the result of Julie's blood test before I met the woman herself. It was a worrying introduction. 'Hb 4.4' was phoned through from the lab. We needed to get hold of her as soon as possible.

Hb 4.4 is a dangerously low haemoglobin reading. Haemoglobin is an iron-based molecule that carries oxygen in the blood. When you have too little haemoglobin in your system you have a blood disorder called anaemia; patients often feel tired or breathless as their organs aren't receiving enough oxygen to function properly. The normal range in women is usually over 11, so Julie was severely anaemic. The most common cause of anaemia is bleeding. For obvious reasons, most people know if they are bleeding, but if you bleed into your bowel, it can be relatively silent. In this situation, you may slowly lose blood into your gut. The main symptoms of anaemia, tiredness and breathlessness, may present themselves, but if they gradually materialise over a few months you may not really notice it. Your body compensates.

This is what had happened to Julie.

It was clearly an emergency. With a reading like this, Julie could become acutely ill at any time. I phoned her mobile and her landline, but both of them rang and rang with no reply.

'I'll have to go round there,' I said to Jonathan. He nodded at once. I jumped in my car and drove to Julie's house. The curtains were drawn back and no lights had been left on. Everything seemed normal. I rang the doorbell, then rang again. No reply.

I quickly called the surgery's main reception desk.

'Look,' I said, 'she isn't answering. I need to get inside – she could be lying on the floor unconscious right now.'

'You're right, Laura. Call the police.'

A situation like this presents a real dilemma. If the police come for a welfare check, there's a very strong chance they'll end up forcing entry to the house.

'But if she's just gone away and she's fine, she won't appreciate coming home to find her front door off its hinges. Is there any other phone number on her record?' I asked.

'Wait a minute,' our receptionist said. 'I've had an idea. I think her mum's a patient here too – and if she is, we'll have her number.'

She was right. When I spoke to Julie's mother, she told me that Julie was away on a retreat and hadn't taken her mobile. She would be back the next day.

Julie was 54 years old and worked in a small niche bookshop nearby. She came into the practice to see me the following afternoon. I explained that her blood test showed a worrying result and that we needed to do some more checks on her.

'Is that really necessary?' said Julie. She seemed to be intelligent and calm. 'Don't worry if I look a bit pale. I'm always pale. I'm sure there's not a problem. I'm only here because I was trying to give blood. When they gave me the iron test, I failed it and they told me to see you. I don't often visit the doctor.'

'I understand,' I told her, trying to keep the anxiety out of my voice. I didn't want to scare her, but she had to understand that this was serious. 'But I really think we should find out what's going on.'

It is rare, nowadays, to meet people who are very ill but believe that they are well. It's usually the other way around. But this was Julie's situation.

'Dr Marshall-Andrews,' she said clearly. 'With no disrespect to you at all, I don't like to follow Western medicine. It only treats the symptoms, not the underlying causes of disease. My sister is a homeopath, and normally if I am feeling under the weather, she prescribes a remedy for me.'

A homeopath? Really? I didn't want to be dismissive, but I didn't think that this was helpful at all. I tried hard to keep a neutral expression on my face.

'I'm sorry, Julie,' I said, 'but this is urgent. I think that your results may be telling us something important. I'd really like to send you for tests.'

Not surprisingly, Julie wasn't happy with the tests I was proposing. Who would want to have one camera pushed down their throat into their stomach and another one inserted through their anus into their colon? But she agreed to be urgently referred for both these procedures.

A large tumour was found at the base of her oesophagus, the tube which extends from the mouth to the stomach. It must have been there for a while, curling around her gullet and oozing blood into her stomach. The word 'cancer' comes from the Greek for 'crab' or 'creeping ulcer', and it is easy to see why this was chosen as a name so long ago.

For Julie, the news kept getting worse. A more detailed scan revealed that the cancer had spread into the liver and lymphatics in her chest. Gently, the oncologist – a specialist in cancer – explained her prognosis. This thoughtful, interesting woman had only months left to live. Her care was handed back to us and the Palliative Care Team. They look after patients approaching the end of their lives.

But when I next saw her, Julie was remarkably upbeat.

'I'd stopped noticing how tired I was feeling,' she said to me. 'I thought it was just my time of life. But those blood transfusions in the hospital made such a difference.'

Julie had been transfused several units of rich, dark blood. As a result, her haemoglobin levels were much higher. In herself, she was actually feeling much better than she had for a long time. I noticed another difference too – it was as though the sudden defining of her life expectancy had given her a clarity and purpose she had not had before. She reduced her hours at work and spent more time with her friends. One weekend a friend drove her to Bristol.

The next time I saw her for an appointment, she was very excited.

'While we were down there, we found the Penny Brohn cancer unit,' she explained. 'I went inside and talked to them – and they were so lovely. They inspired me.'

I looked at her. She was obviously tired and not well, but the energy and enthusiasm in her voice were mirrored in her eyes. Something very nurturing for her had clearly happened in Bristol.

'What did they say?' I asked.

'They understood how I was feeling. They listened. They knew I don't just want to take medicines – that people with this illness need so much more than that.'

Penny Brohn was diagnosed with breast cancer in 1979. She recognised the importance of caring not just for a patient's body but for their 'mind, spirit, emotions, heart and soul'. She and a great friend, Pat Pilkington, got together with a group of volunteers and therapists and founded her centre. Theirs was one of the first instances of Integrated Medicine – a way of caring for patients that sees them as unique individuals, not just as cases, and sets out to meet their emotional needs and those of their families.

Penny Brohn didn't oppose Western medicine. She was an advocate for all the advances it offers, but she also understood the importance of supporting the person themselves, not just focusing on the tumour growing within them. It was clear straight away from the response to her work how many people agreed with her. Her new centre was a big success. Its ethos was later developed and expanded by a woman on her own cancer journey called Margaret Keswick Jenks – the founder of Maggie's centres.

Maggie Jenks was diagnosed with advanced breast cancer in 1993. When she received the diagnosis, she was sitting with her husband in a dingy room in the Western General Hospital in Edinburgh. Her abiding reflections on that moment were that at this most shocking and important time of her life, there was nowhere to collect her thoughts, nowhere to cry and be comforted. And if she felt this way, Maggie realised, so must thousands of others.

So she set about creating and designing a cancer centre where patients could go and be supported, have a cup of tea and a chat, get a massage or some acupuncture. She, like Penny Brohn, wanted to create a gentle, nurturing place that could help heal and restore the damage not just to patients' bodies, but also to their minds, souls and hearts. Maggie died in 1995; over the years more Maggie's centres have emerged alongside other major hospitals that care for patients in this way in the country.

For Julie and for me, the discovery of Integrated Medicine was to be life-changing.

*

When I was a medical student in Southampton, I made the decision that paediatrics – children's medicine – was the path I wanted to take.

I had set my sights set on the lofty heights of becoming a consultant paediatrician at Great Ormond Street Children's Hospital. Working with sick children – sometimes extremely sick, or with life-limiting conditions – sounds draining but in truth can be inspiring and even uplifting; to feel that you can make a difference to people's lives at times of real crisis is a great privilege. Scientifically, the work was fascinating too; I saw cutting-edge research and remarkable advances in children's medicine and felt like I was part of the advance of science in its war on suffering and disease. I attacked my professional goals with energy and passion, achieving membership of the Royal College of Paediatrics and Child Health in record time. I landed a job at the Chelsea and Westminster Hospital and a young, dynamic consultant there took me under his wing. I was on course – I could feel it. I made connections at Great Ormond Street. I started to draw closer and closer to my dream.

And then I had a baby and my whole world changed.

I found that my hunger for the job had died. There was something else that mattered more: a tiny, wriggling, never-sleeping thing – Josh. I struggled on for a few months, stretched between the career I had committed my life to and my new-found love. But I could no longer stay at work until the job was done. I felt the guilt of having to leave while my colleagues carried on, only to arrive late at the nursery and collect the last remaining baby. It was as though I was failing everywhere – I couldn't be the doctor that I wanted to be, or the mother that I wanted to be either. This feeling broke my heart. I knew my life had to change.

So I left the dynamic, high-flying buzz of hospital medicine and began a reluctant conversion to general practice. I secured a training post at a GP practice in Sompting, a small town just outside Brighton. Here, at least, I would only have to work two or three days a week and could get home at a reasonable hour.

I found myself driving through the streets of Sompting to start my first day as a GP trainee early one autumn morning in 2002, and was instantly afraid that I had paid a heavy price for my change in career. Sompting consists chiefly of bungalows – and to my eyes, that morning, they were all grey. The sky was grey, the sea was grey, the houses were grey and the people who moved slowly outside them were also grey.

All of a sudden, it hit me that I had undoubtedly made the biggest mistake of my life. There was absolutely nothing cutting-edge about Sompting. I had walked away from the greatest sense of professional purpose that I had ever known. What was I doing? I started to cry. I could barely see the entrance to the practice, which was to be my workplace for the next one and a half year, but what I could see of it was also pretty grey.

I pulled myself together, composed my face and walked inside. An elderly lady sat behind the desk. She barely looked up as I entered, but motioned me to sit in a chair that looked like it had been the silent repository for every form of bodily fluid and hot beverage known to man. I remained standing and waited for my trainer to emerge. After a short time, the side door opened and a man in his fifties with unruly hair and physics-teacher shoes appeared. His face crumpled into a smile. He looked like he had completely given up on any attempt at smartness. I glanced down at the smooth lines of my Westwood suit. I did not belong there. This was not my place.

My trainer, Dr Benson – Harry – led me to my room.

On the desk, I saw a long box of notes belonging to the patients who were booked in to the morning's clinic. An old computer sat on the corner of the desk, largely unused.

'We are transitioning to a paperless system,' Harry told me. It didn't look like there was much transitioning going on.

'I'm just next door if you need anything! I'll come and get you at coffee time. We all meet for coffee at 10.30,' he said cheerily.

I closed the door and started to cry.

I started up the computer and searched rapidly for NHS jobs. I had to get back into a hospital. This was going to kill me. I felt sure it would be a long, protracted and grey death.

14

While I was looking for a part-time job anywhere else in the world but Sompting, a buzzer sounded. My first patient had arrived.

I picked up her notes. Betty Knowles, eighty-four years old. Grey. I went out and called her in.

Betty was a small woman who appeared surprisingly sprightly for her great age. She had an unusual energy about her as she looked around the room.

She leant forward, drawing me towards her.

'You could make a bit more of this place, darling,' she whispered conspiratorially. I sniffed back the tears and looked around at the little cupboard of a room I was in. A small window looked down on an apple tree outside. Behind it there was a garden with a gnome in it.

'Yes, I suppose I could,' I replied.

She began to explain that she had a pain in her thumb and forefinger which had been there for many years. I could feel utter despair setting in again.

'It's probably from all that sewing,' she commented.

'Did you sew a lot?'

'Oh yes, dear. I was Marilyn Monroe's seamstress.'

'Did you get to know her?'

'Oh yes, sometimes we would chat for a whole afternoon. The things that went on! I saw it all!'

What a fascinating past she must have had, this woman I'd dismissed as dull and grey. In that moment, I understood how my arrogance and my vanity had clouded my vision. We talked about her life, and as I listened, I started to realise that people each have their own stories, and that almost all of these were intriguing. As my next patient came into the consulting room, I managed a welcoming smile, behind which was also a slightly better attitude.

My second patient was four. His name was Johnny. His dad had brought him to see me as he was worried that Johnny's foreskin was too tight.

I asked him what led him to believe this was the case and he explained that his boy's foreskin didn't seem to retract comfortably. I reassured him that any seeming tightness was pretty normal, and usually sorted itself out by the time a boy reached about six years old. In the absence of infections and any problems peeing, I suggested we should leave it well alone.

But Dad was really concerned and wanted me to have a look. Johnny, however, was not so keen.

Dad and Johnny had clearly been debating what Johnny would need to do in this moment for some time. Johnny was already sucking on an enormous lolly – one of those large solid sugar ones in the shape of a dummy.

'Now, Johnny,' his Dad said sternly. 'We discussed this earlier and you said that if I bought you that lolly, you would show this lady your willy.'

Johnny sized up the situation, took a long draw on the lolly and shook his head.

Dad tried again but the response was the same.

'What about if I buy you an even bigger lolly?'

Johnny shook his head, swinging his legs on the chair. This kid will go far, I thought.

I was about to intervene when Dad had a brain wave.

'Will you do it if I do it?' he asked.

Both Johnny and I looked at him. Johnny nodded his head. I remained too stunned to object.

Dad took a deep breath, closed his eyes, stood up and dropped his trousers and pants.

He looked round at Johnny from his grossly compromised position.

'There,' he said triumphantly. 'Now you.'

Johnny looked at him carefully for a second and considered his options.

Then he shook his head.

If this was what being a GP was like, I thought, I would be just as fascinated working here as I was in my time as a high-flying hospital practitioner. My new direction might not be the terrible mistake I'd first feared. I took another glance out of the window at the garden gnome. This time, I thought I saw a twinkle in his eye.

*

Julie came back from the Penny Brohn centre in Bristol with a very clear idea of how she wanted to die. Meaning and purpose are probably the most important features of fulfilled lives. They often come in the form of love and relationships but sometimes, as for Julie, they present themselves as beliefs and ideas. Some people have a sense of meaning and purpose guiding them for many years. They are fortunate. For others, it comes in brief periods, or at the end of their lives.

Julie didn't have much money, but she talked about the types of treatments that she felt would help her. She wanted homeopathy and acupuncture and had found well-qualified practitioners she trusted. Julie and I began a journey as doctor and patient that deeply changed the way I looked at my role.

As the cancer spread throughout her slight body, Julie weakened. The tumour pressed into her spine and lungs, but every time I saw her to review her pain she would decline medication. She had reflexology, acupuncture and massages instead of morphine and, amazingly, for her, it worked. This was the method of her choice. She was calm; she drew friends and professionals around her. But she was also spirited and firm. She argued with the oncologists and Palliative Care Team. She did not want to follow the usual pattern. She wasn't going to be pushed into a clinical pathway.

Instead of feeling frustrated with her, I watched her and tried to help where I could. I understood that often Julie did not come to me because she wanted drug treatment. She wanted reassurance and support.

When she was very weak, Julie decided she wanted to go to the Gower Peninsula in South Wales on holiday. This had been an important place for her when she was growing up, and she had not been back there for many years. Clinically, the trip seemed like madness. She could hardly stand, she was skeletally thin and required help most of the day. The Palliative Care Team were worried she might die there. She would need palliative support while she was away that we clearly could not provide from Brighton.

We spoke to local services in Wales. It was difficult and it required already stretched teams to think outside the box and do something unusual. But in early spring, Julie made it back to the Gower. She was surrounded by friends and family there. It was March but the weather was unusually good. I called her once and she was sitting at a beach-side café overlooking the cove. She had blankets and cups of tea around her as she watched her nephews playing on the beach. There was a steep coastal path, which her brother-in-law had managed to negotiate with her in a chair. They had sat overlooking the sea for some time, high up on the cliffs. Her voice was stronger than it had been for months, fortified by the sunshine, sea air and love.

In the end she had the full works: a syringe driver of high-dose medication and full hospice care. She played cards with the hospice nurses in the evenings right up until her death, and when I visited her there, she was still smiling, although clearly very tired.

'Dr Marshall-Andrews,' she said to me. 'I know you didn't really want to listen to me when I talked about alternative care. But you did, and I very much appreciate it.'

'Oh dear – I thought I'd disguised all my doubts far better than that!'

Julie chuckled.

I could see the peace of mind she had found in her last weeks. If she'd done exactly as she was told and followed the conventional cancer treatment route, the outcome would still have been the same – but for Julie and her family, the journey there would have been so different. That wasn't what she'd wanted to do – and she had the right to choose. She took her own path to death, and showed me that another way existed.

Just one thing was preying on my mind. I'd still not said a word to my practice partner, Jonathan, about the way I was thinking. But I couldn't see any conversation that included the words 'Integrated Medicine' going well. Jonathan was a good GP, a hard-working and sensible man who wanted the best for his patients. But I knew with absolute certainty that he wouldn't be receptive to this kind of thing at all. I decided to keep my ideas to myself for the time being. But I could feel the distance between us growing, as the pull towards a different way of practising medicine grew stronger and stronger in me.

*

Once I'd met Elizabeth, keeping quiet became a lot harder.

I remember her clearly. She was suffering from a lung disease called bronchiectasis, which made her prone to protracted pneumonias, and often led to crippling bouts of depression. But I found I still looked forward to seeing her – her energetic approach to life couldn't help but inspire me. In our consultations, we would talk as much about the ills of the world as about her symptoms and medication.

She was a thickset woman, tough and gritty. She had a gravelly voice and wiry blonde hair that sat stiffly on her head. Her lung disease impaired the flow of air across her vocal cords and she had a constant productive cough. I was surprised when she came to see me one day, full of excitement that she had found the cure for all her sicknesses: singing.

'I've joined a group!' She paused to cough, then excitedly pressed on. 'I've been twice already and I've had the most wonderful time!'

'Singing?' I questioned. I didn't want to sow the seeds of doubt in Elizabeth's mind, but putting more strain on her lungs didn't sound like a good idea.

'I haven't sung for forty years – and quite honestly, I never realised what I was missing!' she went on. 'There are more than a dozen people, and some of them – well, it's really most remarkable. They all say the same – that singing has helped them in all sorts of ways.'

I tried to give her an encouraging smile.

Over the next few months, Elizabeth sang every day in the group she had found. To my amazement, her mood improved, she stopped having to take the antidepressants she so hated and her lung function was much better too. Most winters were treacherous for her. She would spend much of the time on antibiotics and often required hospital admission. But as she sang herself through that winter, she only needed for two short courses of medication. I started to pay more attention to her theory that singing was healing her.

One day, she brought a visitor to see me.

'This is Udita, doctor – the lady who runs our singing group!'

Udita greeted me with a wide, warm smile. She turned out to be a lovely, gentle woman with a softly spoken charm and kindness that made you listen carefully when she talked. And she brought evidence and case studies with her, mainly from the Sidney De Haan Research Centre in Canterbury. These showed convincing models of singing as a huge adjunct to the care of Parkinson's disease, lung disease, depression and anxiety, with many more wide-reaching benefits.

'"Sing for Better Health" makes a really big difference to our members,' she explained. 'We think it's partly physical – it helps the lungs get stronger – but most of all it's the sense of community, of making something beautiful together, that helps people. It takes people beyond themselves, and it's joyous.'

I looked across at Elizabeth, who gave me a grin. Joyous, I thought, was certainly the word. The more she sang, the more her depression seemed to lift, and along with it, her energy levels too. She became an incredible powerhouse of unstoppable passion, hellbent on changing the delivery of healthcare. She adopted me as a willing accomplice and we started on a journey that was to radically change my life and hers. We wanted to create a community of artists, dancers, singers and writers who could help support people through their stories of illness and wellness. We even started to talk about holding a singing group in the waiting room of the surgery.

I was growing more and more excited. It was becoming clear to me that interventions like this could offer a truly holistic treatment for people with very significant disease. They offered not only a measurable impact on physical function, but also a significant improvement in mood and quality of life. For so many people, loneliness can be a limiting issue that also negatively affects prognosis, and social activities such as singing groups seemed to me to be a fantastic solution.

Here was the inspiration I really needed to go forward. I decided I was ready to make big changes in the way I worked, and integrate these new ideas. Non-traditional methods of care made a difference to patients – I could see it very clearly. *Why* exactly this was, I didn't know. I was curious to learn more. The only time that doubt would creep into my mind was when I wondered what Jonathan would think.

Then national politics helped me. That certainly doesn't often happen – but just this once, it did. The Labour government under Tony Blair was passing laws at the time on health and safety regulation for healthcare providers. The problem was that the vast majority of general practices existed (and still do) in old converted buildings like the small converted Victorian house that our practice was situated in. The steep staircases and narrow, oddly-angled doors were hard to negotiate, even for the most athletic among us. In fact, it was not uncommon to see one of us wedged between the door and the wall upon leaving the toilet. The Labour government's new laws aimed to improve accessibility and rapid emergency exits. But old practices could not come close to meeting the new requirements. So there was a big push to re-house a lot of the worst and most inappropriate practices – and our little higgledy-piggledy building was high on the local authority's list.

I felt sure that this potential move for our practice was an opportunity to do something incredible – to go in a whole new direction. Elizabeth was a constant source of ideas and inspiration, and she and I talked about other projects in the local area. She was my relentless detective, finding out innovative programmes and bringing them to my attention. I imagined a practice with large, light rooms and art groups and singing groups and beautiful decoration with inspiring health messaging that offered more sustainable solutions to people's health needs: solutions that did not necessarily involve medication, but that relied more heavily on community and connection and lifestyle change.

Meanwhile, Jonathan and I went to a meeting with a representative from the Clinical Commissioning Group about finding ourselves a new premises. The CCG had been liaising with the council and had found an old church that was for sale. We went to see it.

It was a sunny day and we gathered outside a flint-walled building tucked down a side street off the main high street in Brighton. The lady from the CCG let us in with an enormous key that looked like it must have been at least 100 years old. There was a slightly damp smell – the place must have been unused for some time, patiently waiting for the next burst of energy, life and imagination to be stamped onto it.

I could see straight away that the building was absolutely perfect: it had high ceilings and big rooms, and lots of communal space for groups and events. Jonathan's sister, Sarah, was an architect, and she had come along with us to view the property. I rushed around painting a picture in words of what could be in this dusty old building. Jonathan and Sarah followed me, umming and exchanging glances.

'And in this central bit we could have interactive art installations with positive messaging about behaviour change,' I gushed. 'We could run nature walks and mindfulness-based narrative groups.'

I couldn't stop. It was as though I had verbal diarrhoea. Any moment I was going to burst into song. Elizabeth was going to come dancing in from stage left with her chorus of healed singers, leaping and twirling.

We left and walked back to our practice. I asked Jonathan what Sarah thought of the project. 'Well,' he replied dryly, 'she thinks we have one big problem.'

'Oh no – what's that?'

'You,' he said and walked into his room.

Well – that took the wind out of my sails. I already knew that Jonathan was frank to a fault. I struggled not to take what he'd said personally, but it was hard. In retrospect, though, I'm glad he was so blunt. I knew then that I was going to have to leave. Jonathan and I just weren't on the same page any more. And if you're going to head in a whole new direction, it's vital that you do it with people who have the same vision.

I had to find a new practice. I needed a place that was mine, where I could make this vision a reality.

*

I started to imagine what a truly integrated practice could look like. It would have multifunctional rooms that could be used by therapists and doctors alike. As well as modern medicine, it would offer classes in meditation, mindfulness, nutrition, yoga, singing and more. It would be beautiful, modern, inspiring. This was a heady and exhila-rating time. A colleague and I spoke to politicians and local council members. We identified land on the Brighton seafront and started to explore ways in which the project could be financed. There were times when I could almost feel the texture of the newly moulded walls and smell the final coats of paint. The project was a constant presence in my mind.

It was also, I realised as our planning went on, an absolutely massive undertaking – too massive. With the resources I had at the time it seemed to be a cloud, unreachable in the blue sky. But whenever I started to feel this way, I reminded myself of what it was that I was trying to achieve, and continued to put plans in place that would help me to make everything a reality as soon as the right time came. So a few months later, when the opportunity arrived, I was ready.

*

It was a blustery evening. Squalls of sea-soaked air buffeted the door of the taxi as I stepped out onto the main road that runs along the Brighton coast. The tall Georgian terraced houses that characterise the city stood like sentinels, resolute against the onslaught. This was not new to them. The storm would pass, they would remain. I ran from the car into the large porch of one of the close-by houses. A collection of door bells lined the wall to the left of the door. It's a constant source of amazement to me that at one time these enormous buildings housed single families, probably just for the summer. Now some of them are made up of ten or even twenty flats. That night I was heading right to the top floor, to a doctors' dinner party in a slightly swaying garret flat on Marine Parade.

I don't have many friends who are doctors. This is unusual as doctors often band together – it's safer that way. You are less likely to shock or offend people with your macabre observations or gallows humour. So it's always something of a relief to attend a universally medical social event. I can tell all my awful jokes that would have normal people staring at me in shocked silence or reaching for the vomit bucket.

I arrived into a prettily lit room full of chatter and life, a welcome, warm contrast to the howling gale outside. The talk over dinner that evening was of the Health Secretary Andrew Lansley's sweeping new proposals – more change, more bureaucracy to assimilate and understand, another politician trying to make his mark on the beleaguered NHS. It was a jovial conversation, but there was an undertone of cynicism and exasperation.

I was seated next to a woman called Hilary. She ran a busy practice near to mine, in Brighton city centre. It was in a notoriously difficult area, and she had large numbers of patients with 'complex needs': substance misuse, alcoholism and homelessness. Along with this, Hilary specialised in patients with HIV and gender dysphoria. Her practice partner had just left to move to the relative safety of Worthing, a small town about ten miles along the coast. She was now on her own, the last woman standing on a ship that was very nearly sunk. She was struggling to get locum doctors as the patients she treated were so difficult to manage. I actually knew one of the locums who had given the place a try, and who gaily told me she would never work there again as 'the patients were all *really* ill'. She added, by way of compensation: 'Lots of serious pathology, though. I've not seen that extent of disease outside a textbook!'

Hilary was sixty-six years old and at the end of her working career. She had hung on in an attempt to stabilise her volatile practice. Now, as its last remaining partner, she had boxed herself in. Most GP practices operate as partnerships, so both the contract with the NHS and the lease of the building are held personally by the GPs. So if the practice fails and has to close, it's the GP who has to pay the lease on the building for the remainder of its term. That was the situation Hilary faced. If she left, the practice would fold and she would be left with a ten-year lease on an expensive high-street building.

Hilary had worked tirelessly for many years, but she was rapidly running out of the energy to keep going. Against a background of chat and chinking glasses, she poured out her heart. I could really see how desperate she felt.

'At this stage in my career, it's just too much,' she told me. 'I'm approaching retirement – or at least I should be. It's the lease that's the really big problem. I don't see any way out that doesn't leave me financially crucified.' Tears spiked her eyes. I felt terribly sorry for her. And then as I listened, I realised that there might just be a way to help us both. What if I could find the new direction I was looking for, and allow Hilary the peaceful retirement she so deserved?

The next morning, I ran to work early. Our practice manager, Gary, was already there. He was sitting in the damp basement at his desk, which listed badly to the left – so much so that it was impossible to open the bottom left-hand drawer. Jonathan had a sharp eye for profit and wasn't keen on unnecessary expenditure. A desk with drawers that actually opened apparently sat far outside the realm of 'necessary'.

I flew down the stairs, fired up with the idea that had been percolating in my mind all night. 'Gary, I found a practice! I am going to take over from Hilary! She wants to leave and there are no other partners.'

'What?! You're leaving us, Laura?' he cried. I realised from his shocked expression that my journey of ideas had taken place very much outside work, in my own time and inside my own head. I hadn't shared them with any of my colleagues. Perhaps I'd been afraid of their reactions. But if I was truly going to strike out on my own, I decided, it was time to be brave and go public.

'Yes, Gary. Yes, I am. I want to do patient care differently. I've seen some new methods working already – alternative methods. Don't get me wrong – I'm still a scientist, and scientific rigour is important, but it's only part of the picture. We understand a lot of things about illness, but I think there are things that we don't understand. I want to learn more about these things and how they can help us treat patients. I want to actually put them into practice.'

Gary jumped up as though what I'd said was an immediate call to action. 'I'm coming with you!' With Gary on board I knew the chances of success would be much greater. It gave me strength.

'We can be partners,' I suggested. And that's exactly what happened. Gary became one of the first practice managers in the country to be a partner of a GP practice – and what a brilliant one he turned out to be.

Our little team expanded when we asked our colleague Francis to come with us. He had moved down from a practice in London to live near the sea. When Jonathan and I interviewed him for a position, we found ourselves drawn to his personality. It was clear that he was amazingly intuitive and skilled as well as clever, and nothing less than brilliant with computers. We'd hired him on the spot. From day one, I'd known that we were lucky to have him on board.

I phoned him at home and put the proposition to him: a new, pioneering practice and a fresh approach to medical care. In a rare rash moment, he agreed to come on board. So we three left to start our adventure.

I don't think any of us realised at that stage what we were about to let ourselves in for. I remember a senior GP colleague staring at me wide-eyed and horrified as I explained my plans to her. 'That's very brave of you, Laura,' she said. Bravery is not generally thought to be a good thing in medicine. Doctors tend to be cautious, considered, risk-averse. Many of our colleagues believed that we were taking a pretty big risk.

And, of course, we were.

*

On 1 July 2013, we walked into our new practice. It was a far cry from the spacious modern building on the seafront that I'd imagined, but it was ours and it was real. Gary always says now that if he had known back then just how hard a journey it would be, he would never have undertaken it. I am so glad he didn't know. Neither of us did.

Sometimes I get flashbacks of those early days that are almost reminiscent of post traumatic stress. Starting a new practice is like walking into someone else's house moments after they have left and carrying on with their life just as it was: their furniture in the rooms, their pictures on the walls, their clothes in the cupboards and their food in the fridge. Initially we had to mimic the life of the previous owners before slowly, bit by bit, we could start to effect change.

Our situation was extremely challenging. Just as Hilary had warned me at the dinner party, many of the patients we were seeing had complicated needs. The location of our new practice gave our problems a real edge of intensity. I couldn't say I hadn't been warned.

Brighton is thought of as fashionable and prosperous. But it also has a dark and troubled underside. It's always had a certain eccentricity – in the nineteenth and twentieth centuries, it was quite the place to 'take the sea air', a magnet for royalty and decadent high living. Its beautiful Regency terraces and squares are a legacy of those boom years on the beach. Today, however, they perfectly capture the current Brighton vibe of polar opposites – lives of total contrast that lived cheek by jowl. Some mansions are exquisitely renovated to provide enormous residences for the rich and famous, while others have been subdivided into numerous poky flats and bedsits, and are badly neglected. I had one patient whose deteriorating mental health caused him to slide from the heights of wealth and success into a life of deprivation and struggle – which was simply represented by him moving next door.

Brighton's bohemian culture has drawn artists and writers. The city became a safe haven for marginalised groups. The LGBT community has thrived in its cosmopolitan arms. Clubs and bars as well as galleries and theatre spaces abound. It is said that Brighton is home to the highest concentration of artists anywhere in the country, maybe even the world. But there's a price to be paid for the city's tolerance. It's a mecca for illicit drugs and alcohol. Along with all its colour and flamboyance, Brighton has the highest incidence of suicides and serious mental illness in the country, and one of the nation's highest rates of homelessness. Much of the homeless population is not from Brighton itself; they have slid down the country, ousted from more parochial towns, and finished up by the coast.

Homelessness has a big impact on our practice. Many of our patients live in one of the four big hostels that our building sits between. Some are ex-servicemen. Some are youngsters on the run from abusive and difficult homes. Some are migrants fleeing torture and war. All are traumatised. Into our waiting room comes a complicated tangle of problems that we must try to resolve.

*

The computers were the first thing that had to be overhauled, we decided. A brand new system was installed, overseen by Francis. Next, the building itself required gutting and revamping. We set out to create consulting rooms that were flexible, able to be used by doctors as well as alternative therapists and practitioners. We tried to fill the place with light to create as much a sense of space as possible. We also wanted rooms where groups could meet – for singing, meditation, crafting and yoga classes, and for talks on many subjects relating to health and wellbeing – so that we could offer our patients varied routes towards wellness. The challenge was to make all these changes happen without compromising on patient care, which meant staying open.

So the builders had to work through the night and at the weekends. This made conditions in the daytime very difficult. Gary and I would arrive at 5.30 a.m. on what was basically a building site. We spent the first few hours of each day hoovering, wiping surfaces, reconnecting computers, and on one occasion working out how to re-plumb the pipes under the nurses' sink. By the time we paused for coffee at 7.30 a.m., before the rest of the team arrived, we were filthy. I still remember the feeling of the plaster dust on my teeth. Dust from the night's work continued settling over the course of the day, and we would all arrive home at the end of our shift covered in a light coating of plaster. Putting up with this was a big ask from a team under pressure, who were handling changes to their computer system and an already complex and demanding patient group. We would smile cheerily at the incoming staff and patients, knowing that we needed to keep everyone on board. We were all too aware that many felt apprehensive about our ambitious plans.

Then there was the financial strain of setting up any new project. Renovating our grubby old building required a huge personal loan. We'd planned very carefully – but still, we were heading into the unknown. This put us under great pressure. The stakes felt very high.

But this was a project all three of us passionately believed in. I was convinced that the environment, the scene in which patients and doctors played out their roles, was vitally important to a sense of wellness and calm. Too many GP surgeries and hospitals I had worked in reminded me of Moscow Airport in the 1970s – they were functional, but austere and unloved. With this new surgery, we had an opportunity to put into practice my deep belief that medicine is largely about relationships and support.

People get better faster if they feel cared for and safe. That feeling starts when you walk in the door of a healthcare setting. I wanted our new practice to make people feel valued. I wanted the presentation of the building and the space to say, 'We care about you. We are thinking about what it feels like to be ill and scared while you sit and wait here.' There should be no scrappy bits of A4 paper stuck on broken pieces of abandoned equipment here. Our message was: 'We attend to this building like we attend to you, with love and kindness and competence.'

A practice is all about the people who work there. We knew that right from the start. Most of Dr Hilary's team had stayed to work for us, but we also wanted to bring on board new people who shared our commitment to new approaches. And we knew that asking the existing staff to come on board with our new approaches would be a challenge.

*

Before we began, Gary and I had attended a garden party Dr Hilary hosted for her staff. At this gathering, she'd announced her retirement and our plans to take over the running of the practice. Two of the Reception team and one of the nurses immediately burst into tears. I watched the dynamics of the group. As Gary and I left that evening, we discussed the team we were inheriting.

'It's all about Maureen,' I observed. 'She has the power in the Reception team. They look to her.'

'Agreed,' said Gary. 'And on the nursing side, it's Jacqui, the advanced nurse practitioner. She's basically run the practice until now.'

They were both the sort of women I loved: tough, principled, fun. I was glad to have them there. But this wasn't a straightforward handover. We were going to shake things up, and expect our new staff to step out of their normal comfort zones and trust us. It was a pretty big ask.

'So what we need is their buy-in,' Gary mused. 'How on earth are we going to get that?'

Maureen, Rachel, Charlotte and Gaynor came first. They were the practice's Reception team – old hands at the game, with lots of experience. And it was in Reception that we were planning one of our first and biggest changes to the 'normal' way of doing things.

Our area, with all its problems of homelessness and poverty, had a high number of patients suffering from addictions, including to very strong opiates – a group of highly addictive pain-relieving drugs. Opiate addiction is a huge problem around the world. In many cases, patients were given these medicines before it was understood just how addictive they can be. Opiate addictions continue to be such a problem as it's not easy to ask people living stressful and marginalised lives to go through the painful and difficult process of withdrawal – and providing these people with with support while they detox is also extraordinarily expensive.

Every Friday, a queue of hungry, angry opiate addicts would file in to collect their prescriptions of pain medication. Sometimes they turned up early, or they had already collected them that morning. Sometimes there had been a mistake made by the practice or the chemist, and they didn't get what they were expecting. All this inevitably led to arguments. Nine times out of ten the police would be called, and someone would be carted off to the cells. It was exhausting and anxiety-inducing, to say the least.

That was why our reception desk was stationed behind a screen of clear, toughened plastic. Everybody thought this was vital in protecting the staff from the onslaught of abusive behaviour and posturing. But now we'd decided to change it. We lowered the reception desk and removed the protective screen. We installed soft lighting under its front panel and put up artwork. We took down the signs warning people that there were 'no addictive drugs on the premises'. As well as being a blatant lie, this sign only served as a reminder, bringing the thought of drugs to the forefront of everyone's mind.

When we were done, our reception area looked more like an expensive beauty salon or art gallery than a busy inner-city GP practice. We proudly unveiled the new arrangement one Monday morning. It didn't go down well to begin with. Gaynor, Rachel, Charlotte and Maureen stood staring at us with their mouths open. They were well used to the shenanigans that would regularly occur around their desk.

'You cannot be serious,' Charlotte said. 'We are going to be massacred.'

'I'm not working there,' Gaynor agreed. She was a no-nonsense Scottish woman, tough enough to tell her new bosses frankly what really went on around here. 'It will be carnage. We must have a screen. You'll have to get the builders back.' Somewhat crestfallen, Gary and I agreed. They had moved to another job and would not be available for two weeks. We were just going to have to make do until then.

On the first Friday that the new look was in place, I asked Gary to keep a close eye on Reception. Maureen and Charlotte were on duty, being the most capable at dealing with aggressive patients, but I didn't want the team to feel that their new managers weren't listening to their worries. So Gary seated himself behind the desk, logged on to a PC, and became immersed in work. As the waiting room filled up, he was paying close attention.

Our first opiate user arrived, a man called Trevor, whom we all knew very well. He could be difficult. Charlotte and Maureen, sitting unprotected for the very first time, gave him professionally welcoming smiles, trying not to show that they were nervous. He was obviously startled by the new-look waiting room.

'Morning, Trevor,' said Maureen.

'Ah – morning. I've – ah – come for my script.'

'That's fine. If you can just come over here, we'll have it for you in a moment.'

'What's all this, then?' said Trevor, waving his arms at the paintings.

'It's been smartened up. D'you like it?' Maureen was keeping her voice cheerful.

Trevor surveyed the room.

'It's okay.'

He came up to the desk and stood calmly waiting while Rachel pressed 'print' and his prescription was issued. He was often impatient, but that didn't seem to be the case today.

'Here you go, Trevor,' she said, and slid the script across the open-topped counter.

He picked it up. He took another long look around the room.

'Right then. Thanks. The lights look nice.' And with that, he left.

Something remarkable had happened. It was as if the new environment had drawn out a different type of behaviour. Admittedly, our most hardened street-fighting addicts did not suddenly start wandering idly around the art exhibits, discussing the existential meaning of the works on display... but there was a profound and noticeable change. The 'feel' of the new waiting room created a shift in how people interacted – with us and with each other. The builders never did come back. We only had to call the police out five times in the first six years.

This turnaround gave me confidence. It made me more and more certain that I was right in my core belief – that if we gave dignity to each patient, listened to their feelings and responded to them as an individual, we would all gain so much. I also felt sure this approach would prove cost-effective to the NHS and society as a whole.

Gary shared my belief. He was right there with me, every step of the way. We'd only been working together as partners in the new practice a short time when his mother died, but even though he was deeply affected by grief, he never let it affect his professional focus. He threw himself into his work, maintaining a vibrance and humour that drew people to him, instilling confidence everywhere he went.

Our new nursing team was just amazing. Jacqui, our advanced nurse practitioner, was a competent leader who'd basically been running the whole place for quite a while as Hilary had struggled on alone. She was backed up by Lara, our Polish nurse, a woman buzzing with so much energy that her internal dial seemed to be permanently stuck on HIGH. But she also had a wonderfully dry sense of humour and although she never appeared to stop moving, somehow she still managed to notice the way a patient felt. She was enormously caring and warm.

Then there was 'Mary Poppins' – the name we all gave to the lovely Sue, who worked for the city-wide homeless team. So many of our patients were homeless that she became a regular visitor to the practice. Eventually we offered her a job – just in case the wind changed and she had to go away and not return.

Sue took charge of our nursing visits. Her years of working with the most manipulative and violent people had not jarred her or given her any discernible edge of cynicism. She was always light-spirited, gentle and hugely kind. Our weekly supervision sessions remained the highlight of my week. She was an excellent addition to our team and quickly amassed a collection of adoring housebound patients who waited patiently for her to arrive. She in turn adored them. Brighton's steep hills and tall, narrow houses make prisoners of many people with mobility issues, and mental illnesses like anxiety, paranoia and agoraphobia can build restrictive iron bars around even the most physically fit. Home visiting is vital. It takes a lot of time, but it can truly transform people's lives.

One of Sue's early successes was with a lady called Constantine Littledale. She had uncontrollable diabetes and was on twenty-eight different medications to try to reduce her sugar levels and combat the devastating effect the disease was having on her body. She was constantly on the verge of hospitalisation. The community nurses had been going in for years, trying to work out what was going on. Something must be causing her dangerously high blood glucose levels – but what? They had been through her diet and even surreptitiously checked the fridge. Carers visited three times a day to administer large quantities of medication. But nothing seemed to work. She had us baffled.

Sue went in and started spending time with Constantine. She didn't berate her or judge her, just listened and watched with kindness. Sue noticed that although she had not left her flat for ten years, Constantine insisted on carrying her smart black leather handbag with her at all times.

'Why do you need it?' Sue enquired casually.

'Emergencies!' was the obvious answer.

Then one day, Constantine shared the contents of her handbag with Sue: her passport (fifteen years out of date), five pounds in cash, eight bags of Skittles, five packs of Polos, four packs of Werther's Originals, two packs of Rolos and some indeterminate yet sticky loose items at the bottom.

'How many of these do you eat in a day?' Sue asked innocently.

'All of them,' was the reply.

It turned out that Barry from next door was the culprit: he was bringing the sweets round. He thought he was helping her. Sue gently suggested that the sugar in the sweets might be the reason her diabetes was so out of control. Constantine was genuinely amazed.

'Because of those little sweeties?' she asked. At first she refused to believe it, but with the help of Barry (and sugar-free varieties of sweets), her diabetes is now under control on significantly fewer medications.

Also on our team was Dr Lolita Simcock, an outstanding GP married to one of the most inspirational oncologists of our generation, who had been working tirelessly on protocols around sexual health and HIV. Half-Spanish and half-Leicesterian, she moved with the focus and speed of someone who spent significant time on a spin bike. She was seriously clever – and when it came to rooting out the diagnostic clues in a patient's history, she was like a dog with a bone, refusing to give up until all stones were turned in the search for a patient's troubling symptoms. I deeply admired her tenacity – and over and over again, when specialist consultants organised multiple high-tech investigations to follow up on her suspicions, they would find that she was right. Funny and beautiful, she was also the life and soul of a party.

Lolita bonded brilliantly with Sam, another of our doctors. He had spent most of his career as an anaesthetist, then decided he wanted to move to an area of medicine in which patients were, at least for the most part, conscious. So he'd retrained in general practice. I found him to be solid, kind, and a safe pair of hands. He had a rare combination of emotional insight and tolerance along with a strong sense of justice and equality. Thick, greying stubble covered his chin and his hair was cut close to his head and receding slightly. His bright blue eyes flickered intelligently as he talked. He had a slightly arthritic knee, which gave his stocky body an uneven gait.

Although Sam had always been a man, he was born with a female body and had lived with this dissonance for most of his life. He had had three children before he managed to work up the courage to bring his external appearance into greater coherence with his internal self. Patients would sometimes appear bewildered when he empathised with their stories of labour pain or let slip a personal breastfeeding anecdote. But their bewilderment usually did not last long. This was Brighton, after all – and approximately 2 per cent of our population are members of the trans community. To have a member of that community working as a doctor was a wonderful asset.

We took the decision to employ our own prescribing pharmacist. Shilpa Patel had been working in Superdrug behind the counter when she first met Gary. She had short asymmetric hair and a curious, bright face. She seemed smart, confident and just a bit maverick. In the evenings, with two small children and a pet pig to look after, Shilpa had completed a course so that, unlike most pharmacists, she could both prescribe and dispense medication. She was perfect and she revolutionised our medication monitoring.

We needed her for another reason too. The practice has always been under pressure to save money, as all NHS trusts are. We get regular bulletins asking us to change everyone's brand of asthma inhaler to a cheaper one, or everyone's diabetic medication to something more affordable. It takes a lot of time, and it causes confusion. Patients, especially the elderly, don't like it as their medication suddenly looks different. Their blue pill is now red. 'Change this drug', 'don't use that drug', 'now use it again'. I wonder how cost effective all this really is when you add up all the hours doctors spend managing changing medication requirements. Especially when they could be spending that time seeing patients. I also wonder about the unknown harm it does to patients who misunderstand their medication.

Prescribing in general practice has therefore become highly complex. More and more people are discharged from hospital services on ten or more medications, which need careful monitoring and review. Each medication may require that the patient has frequent blood tests to check kidney function, mineral levels or white blood cell counts. A person's change in weight or blood pressure may affect their dose regime. It's complicated. And it's dangerous. Estimates of deaths related to medication errors range between 1,700 and 22,000 a year in the UK alone.

Shilpa and our new in-house team took all of this on board. They ran safety checks, changed medication, and monitored dosages. We now have three pharmacists at the practice working under her expert guidance and tutelage. They comb through medications, looking for errors and adverse drug interactions. They run audits and develop processes and procedures. Shilpa's work is vital to everything we do.

But there was more to the new practice than prescriptions. We were there to do things differently. Slowly and carefully, we began to introduce the team to its newest members, upstairs in the Wellbeing Suite, smelling of geranium and lavender.

The therapists.

With them came the sense that something genuinely different was happening. But there were also, inevitably, some feelings of suspicion and apprehension. Who were these new people, and what were they going to be like? How would their presence change the status quo?

*

Ben was an acupuncturist who headed up a nearby holistic health clinic at the time. I'd heard about his work through Elizabeth. Born in New York, he'd come to the UK after completing his acupuncture training, and met his British wife on a retreat in the Cotswolds. He was clever and well educated. He was calm and smelt of wheatgrass and something fermented.

I invited him to join our practice, where he would head up our new team of therapists. We decided it would be good for them all to join our fortnightly clinical meetings.

I arrived slightly late for the first joint meeting to see the therapists occupying one half of the room, surrounded by health snacks and coconut water, and the clinical team the other half, eating Quality

Street that were donated by a grateful patient. When I asked Ben to say a few words about the work that he did, there were nods and smiles of welcome around the table. Underneath, though, I could tell there was a pretty heavy dose of scepticism. Ben obviously sensed it – though I noticed that he didn't seem too fazed. He must have been used to this response when he met doctors – and he'd clearly decided on the best way to tackle it.

'So,' he said, 'Laura's interested, and Gary's prepared to come on board – but what do the rest of you really think about acupuncture?' He aimed the question at the medical side of the table, which was definitely becoming restless.

There was an uncomfortable pause. Then Jacqui ventured a response.

'It's not that it doesn't work for some people. I'm sure it can help,' she said politely. There was something in her voice that suggested she wasn't sure at all. 'It's just that a lot of the patients we see are *really* ill. They aren't, well – just slightly anxious middle-class people. It's much easier to help those. Our patients here are properly sick.'

Ben thought for a moment.

'Right, I get it. Why don't you give me some of your really sick patients? I'll see them for free. I won't ask them to change any medication, obviously, but let's just see what happens. Only if the patients are up for it, of course.'

Jacqui considered her options. Her face was intent as she scrolled through a list of names in her mind. Then a slow, triumphant smile crept over her face. 'Terry Clark.'

'Ha!' Lara exclaimed loudly. She was unable to contain her glee at this choice of patient.

'I would be happy to see Terry,' said Ben calmly. 'Is there anybody else?'

'How about... Sarah?' I suggested. Sarah was the patient who had once tried to strangle me – it would be a challenge for him, but I believed that if he could help her, then the rest of the team would accept the value of his work.

'Is she back home from Millview, Laura?' Gary asked.

'Yes – she came back a few weeks ago.'

The gauntlet was down. Jacqui would ask Terry Clark and I would ask Sarah if she wanted a trial of acupuncture.

As the team filed out of the room, Jacqui and I hung back to tidy away the plates and glasses of water.

'What do you reckon Sarah and Terry will say?' I asked her.

'They'll say, "Not a chance!"' Jacqui laughed. She looked down at the plate in the middle of the table. There was a leftover date ball sitting there all alone. Ben had brought them along to the meeting. Jacqui picked it up and popped it into her mouth, then grimaced at the unfamiliar taste. She worked quite hard to force it down her throat.

'I still prefer a custard cream,' she joked, and left the room.

Two weeks later we reconvened. This time, I'd made sure I was there early, and tried to instigate a more integrated seating arrangement. It hadn't really worked: there was still the sense of face-off between two sides – a real feeling of tribalism. There was also a gleam of anticipated victory on the medical side. They were relaxed, leaning back in their chairs. They knew what was coming. Or at least, they thought they did.

We started the meeting. Sarah, Ben reported, had initially refused point-blank to see him – but then, out of the blue, she had called up just the day before to change her mind. Her appointment was set for next week.

We moved on to Terry Clark.

Terry was one of our diabetic patients. He was of medium height, with pale, watery blue eyes. He had thinning, light brown hair and was very overweight. He always brought us bags of pick 'n' mix sweets from the unfortunately positioned sweet shop near his house. I suspected he was a frequent customer of theirs, and also of the Domino's

Pizza next door. Terry's blood sugars had been unbelievably high for twenty years, and no amount of persuasion or strict messaging from the nurses had any effect on him. The corrosive sugars circulating around his body had hardened and narrowed his blood vessels and left him almost blind and with very little feeling in his feet, which were covered with permanent ulcers. As is the case with many diabetics, the reduced sensation in Terry's feet was accompanied by a persistent burning pain. We had struggled to resolve this, despite the thirty-eight medications he was taking.

Two years previously, Terry had had a devastating stroke in our toilet and been resuscitated by Jacqui. This was a remarkable achievement given the smallness of the toilet and the largeness of Terry. He had spent two months in an Intensive Therapy Unit (ITU) and then been discharged back into our care – and, by extension, the open arms of the sweet vendors and pizza parlours. The stroke had left him paralysed on his left side. He also had difficulty talking. He spoke slowly, slurring his words as though his tongue was an enormous, unruly element that he was constantly having to control.

The concept of acupuncture was clearly completely new to Terry, but he had agreed to it happily enough and showed up at the appointed time. All eyes now turned to Ben.

Ben took out some A4 papers and laid them out on the table in front of him.

'Well,' he pronounced, 'in traditional Chinese medicine, Terry is suffering with Damp.'

For a moment there was silence and then Jacqui collapsed forward onto the table. It took a moment to realise from the shaking of her shoulders that she was in fits of laughter. Every so often she would try to draw a deep breath and compose her face, but she couldn't stop and carried on uncontrollably convulsing. Her eyes were streaming with tears and it took four tries at least before she managed to speak.

'Oh my God – that's brilliant!' she managed to blurt out before dissolving again into fits of hysterics. 'The thing is, the thing is... that's perfect! Damp is exactly what he is!'

I knew what she meant. Shortly after his stroke, I had visited Terry at home. He lived in a dark basement flat, high up the hill in one of the sprawling estates that extend above Brighton. I walked down the concrete steps that led to the basement door. Despite being built relatively recently, the cement was cracked and uneven. Moss had grown thickly at the edges and started to spread across the whole width of the bottom steps. Clumps of weeds had sprouted from the cracks and mingled with the moss and fungal growths that were thriving in this dingy recess.

I knocked on the door and waited patiently while Terry made his way laboriously down the corridor. He was half-dressed and there was a light sheen on the flaccid skin that hung loosely off his torso. He attempted a small, apathetic smile. Depression and neglect hung in the air; I could feel their cool fingers on the back of my neck. In the dim half-light, it seemed almost as though I was visiting a creature at the bottom of a pond.

Yes, I thought now, as I sat at the table. Definitely Damp.

Jacqui had managed to pull herself together. Ben was explaining his approach.

'Terry will require a course of acupuncture to release the blocked *qi* and enable the fluid and energy flow of his body to be re-established. That will return normal function to the *zang-fu* organs. He needs warming up – a bit of fire.'

That was it – Jacqui was off again. Ben just smiled to himself. I was impressed with his confidence if nothing else.

After the meeting, I felt sure that something had struck us all. There was a definite truth to the diagnosis, despite it sounding so strange; it was like peering into an alternative universe where the houses and the people and trees were all the same – but everything was understood differently and named a different thing. The world was both familiar and unnervingly foreign at the same time. I found myself praying that Terry would find his fire, for all our sakes.

But over the next few days, the divide between doctors and therapists continued to prey on my mind.

'They don't get on,' I said to Gary. 'The Damp thing helped a bit – but basically, it's Therapists versus Medics. They feel like they're playing for different teams. We have to do something to change it.'

'We need to show both teams that the opposition are still nice people,' he suggested. 'Give them a chance to get to know each other.'

'You're right,' I said. 'So – how about a party?'

It is my firm belief that humans are born to party. It's in our blood. It certainly worked in this instance. We hired a nearby bar and a DJ and to my great relief, everyone came. I remember standing at the bar looking back, seeing receptionists talking to acupuncturists and the nurses laughing with the osteopaths. Suddenly we were all just people, doing what people do.

It wasn't easy – but there was a future in all this. I was sure of it. All we needed was to give each other a chance.

*

If acupuncture could help Sarah, I thought, it would be hard for anyone to deny that what Ben brought to the table was significant. We'd certainly put him up against it. As I thought about this, I felt a sudden pang of apprehension. What if he decided it was all too hard? It would be totally understandable if he packed up and headed back to the calm serenity of the leafy Hove suburbs.

He started seeing Sarah every week. I doubted she'd return after her first appointment, but she did. When the team asked Ben for his reports on her, he explained that she was suffering from excessive liver fire and blood stasis from her previous complex trauma as a child.

'I've been working on opening the inner and outer gates and encouraging free flow of *qi* energy,' he told us enthusiastically. 'We are looking to harmonise her body and her spirit.'

I must have looked a bit nonplussed, and others round the table very definitely did.

'In your language,' he continued, 'we are looking at calming her anxiety by enabling her body to release the tension she is holding from her previous trauma. It's that that is driving her condition.'

I nodded. 'It makes sense. As long as I don't try to map what you're saying onto my understanding of the body, it makes sense.'

Ben smiled. 'There is a deeper wisdom in Chinese medicine,' he said. 'It's not just about the chemistry of the body. It's about the energy of the body too.'

A month or so later, I bumped into him in the corridor.

'How's Sarah now?' I asked him.

'She's still an unwell woman. But she's sleeping better, and she's reduced her lorazepam from 5mg to 1mg.'

'Wow,' I said. 'That's really something. Okay, then – keep on treating her.'

Then one afternoon, I popped down to the kitchen to make a cup of tea. I put the kettle on and waited for Gary to come out of his office. He usually did when he heard me come down the stairs. It was a good opportunity to catch up on the day's events so far: a snippet of good news or a vent of frustration.

I was used to seeing a big red tin of the world's cheapest coffee next to the kettle, and an even bigger box of teabags with the name of a supermarket and 'economy' on the side. But now something had changed. There was a selection of interesting herbal teas. Their pretty coloured boxes stacked against the wall formed an intricate mosaic. I made myself a lemon and ginger. Gary arrived.

'Coffee?' I asked him.

'I've stopped drinking caffeine,' he said brightly. 'I really feel fantastic. Ben put me onto it.'

'That's great,' I said. 'And look at all these teas! This is so much better – let's keep doing this.'

At that moment Lolita arrived, bringing a burst of energy with her.

'Laura!' she cried. 'Laura – you will not believe this!'

'Believe what?'

'I've just seen Sarah in the waiting room. She looks amazing – well, amazing for her. I think she's brushed her hair.'

'Good heavens.'

'And she's sitting and waiting – just sitting and waiting. She's not agitated at all. She looks – well, she looks… calm.'

We all three stood, considering this.

'Do you think it could be Ben's acupuncture?' Gary finally suggested. There was a pause.

'I don't know,' I replied. 'Maybe.'

Lolita threw her head back and laughed.

'Who knew?' she said. 'I mean – *who knew*?'

And with that, she loaded five spoons of instant coffee into her cup and headed back to her office.

I saw Sarah for myself shortly afterwards. She still had a fine tremor and tended to react unpredictably to innocuous comments, but there was a definite change in her mood and temperament. Whether this was down to a natural turn of events, or whether it was the acupuncture, I honestly don't know. But she was calmer and more focused and her lorazepam use was significantly reduced. Shilpa was delighted and extremely surprised.

It would be interesting to see how things panned out in the long term. For the time being, though, it was Ben and acupuncture: 1, medical doctors: 0.

*

Our practice emerged like a newborn calf, staggering and spluttering as it found its feet, but gradually, our new creation steadied itself and gained confidence. Everything was starting to take shape.

One evening as I got home from work, I heard loud sobs coming from the kitchen. My middle son, Danny, had taken a tumble. He had a nasty scrape on his arm, and my husband was attempting to apply antiseptic cream. Danny, however, was very clear about who the medical expert was in the family. The moment I walked in, he tried to pull his arm away from Daddy.

'Mummy! Please make it go away, Mummy!'

I grinned at my husband and took over tending the wound. Danny was soon to be disappointed, as he realised that his faith in my Doctor Who-like superpowers of human tissue regeneration was unfounded.

'Dan-Dan,' I said to him, 'I don't think I can do that. But you can! All we need to do is keep it clean and dry, and your clever little body will heal all by itself.'

Over the next few days, we watched it do just that. The raw, bloody area slowly dried and fibrinous strands began to draw his wound together. New skin cells crept in from the outer margins like a soft, protective blanket being laid carefully down.

The process was familiar, but suddenly it seemed as though I was seeing it for the very first time. Healing is a process. It needs to be enabled rather than controlled or forced. If we remove the inhibiting factors of infection – trauma or chronic stress, for example – our bodies and our minds will always try to heal themselves.

*

Terry Clark had complex problems – problems that the practice had struggled with for years. As the months went by, I began to wonder if it was fair for us to ask Ben to make everything come right, and to label him, and acupuncture, a failure if he couldn't.

Ben had told us he would help Terry find his fire. But Terry's body had suffered greatly under prolonged attack from his damaged soul. The early and sustained abuse he had suffered through his childhood had scarred his mind. He believed himself worthless and distrusted most people around him. He had encountered a number of psychiatrists on his journey through life and had picked up a few psychiatric diagnoses along the way. These included dependent personality disorder, depression, and anxiety. His trauma had been noted many times, but never really confronted or dealt with. As a consequence, Terry had locked it away, deep in the dark, impenetrable vaults of his being. However much he tried to forget about it, or keep it hidden, its poison leached into his self-esteem and his ability to love.

As a young man, he replicated the neglect others had shown him by neglecting himself. He ate and drank heavily and smoked constantly. He carried despondency and despair with him like dead weights, making activity and change almost impossible. Our response had been to load him with medication and urge him to change his lifestyle. But these had been ineffective, peripheral tweaks. They didn't stand a chance against the destructive power emanating from the chambers of his past.

And yet, after a year of seeing Ben, Terry was in the best shape that I had ever seen him. He had managed to stop the opiate medication for his painful feet, and it was good to see how this had brightened his personality. And his eyes were no longer deadened by the morphine. Instead, within them I caught the barely perceptible flicker of a fire, somewhere deep inside. Whatever Ben had done to Terry physically, it seemed that he'd warmed a cold, forgotten place where change had been hard to imagine.

Terry joined an LGBT choir that took place near his house – not because he was gay but because his friend went there. The group was welcoming and it turned out that Terry was a pretty gifted tenor. His diabetes went from 'virtually incompatible with life' to 'moderately out of control'. His blood pressure improved and he stopped using his electric scooter as much to get around. These slow, small steps took years to come about – but the trajectory of his disease progression had definitely changed for the better.

Traditional Chinese medicine and homeopathy pay close attention to the personality of a patient in a way that Western medicine absolutely does not. This is despite the fact that chemical reactions that happen in our bodies are hugely influenced by our thoughts and emotions – because thoughts and emotions have physiological impacts. What we think and feel changes the biochemical environment we exist in. So, in reality, our personalities, and emotional states, matter greatly to our health.

Therapists and artists have taught me that, in order to help someone, you need to take a step back and look at everything that's happening to them and around them, not just at their symptoms of disease. And that insight, I believe, is their power.

As Lolita Simcock had asked with a laugh that day in the kitchen – who knew?

*

I went into the practice one Saturday morning not long after seeing Terry to catch up on some admin. The sun was coming through the meticulously cleaned, full-length windows, fresh flowers sat on the reception desk under a jolly rainbow-coloured 'welcome' sign, and the singing group, twenty people strong, was belting out 'Yellow Submarine' with full force in the waiting room.

Elizabeth, who first made me aware of all the medical benefits of singing, had raged against 'the system' right up until her lung disease finally overwhelmed her. I realised it was probably her rage that had kept her alive.

Just before her death, she'd sent me a card from her hospital bed. I opened it after she had died. A friend handed it to me with tears in her eyes. 'She wanted you to have this,' she said softly. I anticipated a note of heartfelt thanks, a tribute to the importance of our relationship.

The note said: 'Don't forget about dementia. They need it too.'

There was another word underneath that I couldn't make out. The writing was spidery, written with a weak hand. Elizabeth had been concentrating on what was most important, right up to the end.

As the strains of 'Yellow Submarine' reverberated through the practice that morning, I felt that a powerful baton of activism had been placed in my hand. I was determined to run with it well.

CHAPTER 2

Here comes Big Pharma

It was early evening. The practice was silent. I walked through its clinical rooms and found something calming, almost restorative, about being alone in this stilled space. After everyone is gone and the door is closed, the practice is peaceful. It's a no-man's land, awaiting the onslaught of the new day.

I sat down in the waiting room on one of the chairs that Gary and I had spent so much time choosing. They are that clear plastic variety, created with vibrant colours and resembling solid jelly. Some of them even have glitter running through them. Gary certainly lives up to the stylish gay stereotype when it comes to interior decoration. The colours of the chairs are taken from our practice logo, a square of Damien Hirst-type dots, painted by Jude, my artist friend.

Jude started the Wellbeing Gallery, an important aspect of life in the practice. The gallery is really the waiting room, but we've tried to make it far more than that. When I asked Jude if we could use her painting as the logo of our new practice, she readily agreed, on one condition: 'Just don't *over-dot* it, Laura,' she said. I promised her I definitely wouldn't.

So, I feel I should take this opportunity to publicly apologise to Jude for thoroughly *over-dotting* the entire place. There are huge multi-coloured dots on all the doors, the internal signs, and a large array of them are back-lit above the entrance. These dots are better than Damien Hirst's, in my opinion. Each one has several colours in it, like little individual worlds. To me, they represent the many varied and individual people we serve.

We had started a Wishing Wall in our waiting room. Long strings of washing line hung across the main whitewashed side wall. A large tub of plain-coloured rectangles of card, with string tied through a hole like gift tags, stood on the floor at the foot of the wall. A banner across the top asked people to 'hang your wishes on our Wishing Wall'.

Within a very short time, there were hundreds of wishes.

'I wish I was thinner.'

'I wish the NHS would never be privatised.'

'I wish I had a car.'

'I wish my daddy was out of prison.'

'I wish I could fly.'

'I wish I could see my mum just one more time.'

I knew that last one had been placed there by the practice manager, Gary.

Our wall was just one small way to show our patients that everybody matters. That each individual voice would be heard. I believe that this is critically important. And yet, it isn't always the case. Instead, the way we treat people in our society has been overtaken by an obsession with evidence-based medicine.

For a long time, doctors have been trained to only value trials that have been conducted on hundreds of thousands of people. In order to ensure that results are accurate, no one taking place in these trials know whether they are receiving real medication or a placebo; they are known as blind trials. And, of course, such trials can only be done on treatments that look the same – a pill or an injection. While evidence is extremely important, the requirement to have these trials means that, often, very valid treatments are overlooked. You cannot 'blind' people to the fact that they are in a singing group or having acupuncture treatment. You can only do these types of trials on drugs.

And big trials also cost big money. Who's got the money? The multinational pharmaceutical companies, collectively known as Big Pharma. It's not in their interest to trial exercise, say, as a treatment for hypertension. Big Pharma can't make money from exercising and singing in the treatment of high blood pressure. So the 'gold standard' treatments – the ones backed up with big data – are usually drugs. If anything else is suggested as a treatment, we hear 'but there's no evidence for that'.

All that really means is: the trials have not been done. But 'there's no evidence for that' is frequently used to mean: it's dangerous – unknown. So don't suggest a singing group. Prescribe an antidepressant. There's evidence for those.

Mass trial data takes years to complete. Even then, the conclusions only tell us how the majority of people in the trial responded. There will always be exceptions. As a doctor, I have no way of knowing if the patient in front of me will respond well to the treatment or not.

I'd asked my first GP trainer about all this, back in Sompting:

'We tell the patients they'll feel better in, say, five to ten days. But some of them feel better straight away, and others never seem to respond. Why on earth is that?'

I still remember the way that Harry chuckled. 'Everybody's different!' he said. That answer didn't really satisfy me, so I questioned other, older medical colleagues. They all said the same thing. There was a chasm of difference between the medicine I had studied, with its reams of literature searches, trials and national protocols, where medication would lead to a result, and the actual way that medicine worked.

When we only care about big data, anyone who's different gets ignored. We take no notice of any patient who doesn't react in a completely standard way. We even feel annoyed with them for not behaving in the way we expect. We stop listening. We stop caring.

When a big research trial is carried out, the number of people involved is called N. When N is many thousands, the results of the trial will be taken seriously. But in my opinion, whether N=1, or N=hundreds of thousands, what the patient says always matters. I was certain that we had to listen to every individual.

*

I remember the very first time I ever made a judgement call that put me in opposition to 'the normal, accepted way of doing things'. Looking back, perhaps it was a sign of what was to come. I'd never quite fitted into the traditional medical mould. Perhaps it had only ever been a matter of time before I rebelled against it.

The patient's name was Philip. I met him when I was asked to sign a legal paper to section him. 'Sectioning' is an abbreviation for detaining someone in a hospital against their will under one of the Sections of the Mental Health Act of 1983. Most often, people who experience psychosis do so for a short, extreme and usually pretty devastating amount of time. Then they come crashing back into reality, like someone who has temporarily inhabited another dimension and then gets beamed back to earth. This can be terrifying. All too often, the reality the patient left behind has changed considerably when they re-enter it. In many cases, their house is trashed, and their friends eye them suspiciously. One of my patients who'd experienced psychosis discovered his bank account on zero and himself the proud owner of a brand-new Bentley, despite the fact that he had never learnt to drive.

For others, however, psychotic beliefs develop over long periods of time. These people are usually resistant to anti-psychotic therapy. They have truly crossed over into a parallel universe from which they are never to return. This was true of Philip.

I was asked to see him with a very senior consultant psychiatrist and the local AMHP (accredited mental health practitioner). We needed to assess whether or not Philip required admission to the local psychiatric hospital under Section. Psychiatric hospitals often have names like Millview or Sunnybank. They are usually far from being as nice as their names imply.

Philip was a small, devoutly religious man from Paraguay. He was Catholic and believed that God spoke to him through various mediums, but only under very specific circumstances. He lived on the other side of town, not far from my home. There had been a number of complaints made to the council about Philip. Most of these had come from his downstairs neighbour, Jean.

Jean was in her mid-fifties. She lived a quiet and respectable life. She almost certainly put her hair in curlers every night, and undoubtedly changed her bed linen and apron on a daily basis. She had very clear ideas about how things should be done, and reported that Philip frequently accessed his flat wearing an aluminsed fire-protective suit. When he wasn't wearing the suit, he would hang it from his balcony, which was unfortunately stationed directly above Jean's kitchen window and created a somewhat alarming view for her.

Getting into Philip's flat posed some logistical problems because, according to God, if we were not wearing one of these suits we were not supposed to enter or leave the flat through the front door unless some fairly specific conditions were met. Sadly, neither I, the consultant, nor the AMHP therapist had access to a suit, and none of us fancied the prospect of rotating in and out of Philip's in order to gain entry. After lengthy negotiations, it was agreed that we could enter in our standard clothing. We would, however, have to ensure that we did not violate the natural order of Philip's flat that was so clear to him, but so hard for anyone else to see.

Philip asked us to remain in a corner of the room by the door; the floor was covered in tinfoil with scratched markings on it. We squished in with our suits and briefcases, pushing up against each other.

Philip was sitting by an altar in the corner of the room, praying. The room was clean but quite odd. There were piles of objects – books and saucepans, among other things – covered in tinfoil positioned around the room. There was nothing casual or absent-minded about the arrangement of the items. The saucepan that sat on three books had its handle pointing at a carved elephant, which was looking at the altar. A pair of red Nike Air Zoom Pegasus Trainers stood on top of three boxes in the middle of the room. On the floor around the boxes lay a ring of feathers.

After a few moments of us shifting uncomfortably in our confined space, Philip turned to us, smiling and relaxed. The AMHP in front of me, whose back was pressing into my doctor's bag, took this as a sign that we could relax our positioning. He went to step forward.

'Don't move,' said Philip quickly and calmly, and he turned back to his praying. Another five minutes or so went by, and I began to feel the cold prickle of sweat on my back. The room was stuffy, and I wondered what would happen if I fainted. When Philip turned to face us again, we stayed rigid in our designated space. The consultant began asking Philip about his day. Philip was polite and kind, humouring the intruders in his room. A discussion about his unorthodox habits commenced and Philip, clearly used to such questioning, patiently went through his reasoning as if talking to very, very stupid people.

'God is complicated, but that is not his fault,' he smiled knowingly. He held a cross on a chain in his hand, which he turned carefully backwards and forwards as he talked, as if sending a semaphore message to an unseen observer. Two turns to the left and one to the right – 'sorry, God, now I have to deal with some more imbeciles.'

Clearly and calmly, he explained the complex reasoning behind not being able to leave the house unless he was wearing a suit. It all rested on how many cars had passed the top corner of the road before two of the parked cars were moved. If it was an even number it was okay, and he could enter and exit the flat wearing normal clothing. If it was an odd number, then it had to be the fire-protective suit. There were many other stipulations that had to be met during the day. On the way to the shop, if a car passed him coming up the hill before he reached the first lamppost, he would have to run as fast as he could down the road, turn left, then double back and touch the green telecom box on his way. If he did not do this, humanity would suffer the consequences. It was his job to keep us all safe.

It was complicated.

When questioned about Jean, and whether he understood that hanging fire-protective suits outside of her kitchen window might upset her, he replied that he saw her point of view, but she would understand him if she knew what he knew. The consultant psychiatrist, the AMHP and I said our goodbyes and stood outside the block of flats discussing the moral and ethical issues of Philip's situation. For him, intricate details and a complex web of meanings and perceived consequences were consistent and interconnected. He was one of only a few people who could see what was happening in his own mind, and he also saw the great dangers of what might go wrong if certain patterns of behaviour were not followed. He was saving us all from damnation and retribution with his tireless and exhausting monitoring. He was never asked to hurt anyone, or hurt himself, by God or anyone else. He believed in peace and calm and these rituals helped to keep order in the world.

The local council wanted Philip sectioned. He was disturbing the peace and upsetting Jean. However, we all agreed that he was not a danger to anyone or himself. We also knew that he was very unlikely to respond to medication. The consultant wondered about electroconvulsive therapy, which is still used in some very severe mood disorders, and some psychotic depressions. But Philip was not showing any signs of mood disorder – he was simply living in a world of different meanings and phenomena. On the other hand, Sectioning him would mean forcibly removing him from his flat. Police officers would have to restrain him and take him to Millview, a place without attractions that certainly does not overlook a mill. There he would most likely be forced to take medication, or injected with medication if he refused. He would possibly have electrodes applied to his scalp and his brain electrified.

I understood that for Jean, Philip and his odd behaviour must be rather unnerving, and that having what was essentially a tinfoil effigy swinging from side to side outside of a kitchen window could be off-putting. People were not supposed to leave their flats in fire-protective suits when there was no fire and run around the estate touching telecom boxes. I had to wonder, though, if she was actually scared of him, or if she just didn't like anything out of the ordinary.

The consultant thought we had no choice. It was unacceptable to behave in the way that Philip did. He was clearly delusional. He held out the Section paper for me to sign. It's a legal requirement that two doctors and an AHMP authorise the decision.

But I didn't agree.

I kept thinking of the fragile order of Philip's flat. Of the potential trauma of his incarceration. There was nothing going on here, I thought, that warranted it.

'Can't the council move Jean? Or find a flat for Philip where his suit won't bother anyone?' I asked.

'They are both refusing to move,' the consultant replied. His tone was curt. He pursed his lips and lifted his chin as if preparing for a fight. His voice was forceful and authoritative when he spoke.

'Come on, Laura – we need to get this done. It's not a pretty business, but there is no other way.'

I had never disobeyed a consultant before that day. But I couldn't sign it. I wouldn't be part of this decision. I knew they would just get another doctor to do it, but it wasn't going to be me.

Philip was sectioned a few days later. Wherever he went after his stint in Millview, it wasn't in our catchment. His notes were transferred out of the area. I felt sad that I hadn't been able to stop that happening.

Doctors need better access to ethical support at short notice. Impartial philosophers or ethicists could help us work through tough decisions like these.

Here was yet another aspect of medicine that medical school training barely equips us for, I thought. It's a hard thing to teach, but not being 'normal' doesn't make you bad or dangerous. Instead of identifying what harm Philip was doing – none at all, in my opinion – and basing our response on that alone, we had conformed to a rigid way of thinking about 'normality'. This was at a grave cost to his wellbeing. I felt that we should have done better.

Our decisions should be based on people's needs, not processes, or the profits of Big Pharma. This was definitely the direction I had always wanted to travel.

Although I didn't know it at the time, this approach was going to get me into trouble.

CHAPTER 3

N=1

One morning as I walked to work, I saw a man running towards me wearing an aluminised fire suit and red Nike trainers. Down the road he came as fast as he could, turning left at the end and then doubling back, touching the green telecom box on his way; it was Philip, keeping us all safe.

I wondered what he had gone through in Millview. Whatever it was, it clearly hadn't changed him. There was nothing more I could have done for him, but it was hard to shake off the nagging sensation that I had let him down. When another patient, Karen, started to see me repeatedly, the same feeling started to grow.

Karen had been an actress in a number of West End plays, and starred in long-running performances of *Cats* and *Annie*. She had long blonde hair and blue eyes, which she accentuated with dark kohl eye liner and lash extensions. Karen was suffering with what appeared to be a complex and partially diagnosed illness. She had extreme fatigue and brain fog, she couldn't sleep and her muscles ached. She had virtually stopped walking and was largely only able to move around with crutches or the support of her husband, a devoted ex-policeman, who worked hard to support her increasing care needs.

She was suffering from a form of hypothyroidism – which is caused by having too low a level of the hormone thyroxine in her body and can have awful effects: tiredness, brain fog, weight gain and a constant feeling of cold. As levels go on dropping, they cause hair-loss, dry skin, heavy periods and infertility. Luckily, most cases of hypothyroidism respond well to a medicine called levothyroxine, a synthetic version of thyroxine.

I reassured Karen that her treatment should be straightforward. Thyroxine is found in the body in at least two forms: the relatively inactive but stable T4, and the highly active but less stable and shorter-acting T3. In most people, T4 can be converted by the body into active T3. So we give T4 to patients in a tablet form. Patients can convert this to T3, and their symptoms resolve.

But this did not happen to Karen. Regardless of the T4 that we were giving her, her blood levels of thyroxine and its allied hormones would not respond normally. Many months went by and her symptoms were no better. I grew more and more puzzled and concerned. I didn't realise then that my efforts to help her would place me on a collision course with the Medicines Management Team (MMT).

The work of the MMT is important. It is part of our local Clinical Commissioning Group (CCG) and formed of a group of pharmacists and administrators, and led by a GP. The MMT has one mission: to reduce the amount that the local NHS spends by lowering the CCG's outgoings on drugs. But this mission does not take into consideration the fact that reducing a practice's expenditure on drugs does not always support ill-health, and therefore risks costing the tax payer more in the long run. I truly believe that if the mission was instead 'to help reduce the taxpayers' overall financial burden in supporting ill-health' doctors could be given a lot more agency to make nuanced considerations when prescribing drugs to our patients, and therefore be better able to support them.

The MMT heavily scrutinises our prescriptions, and we are required to show and explain our prescribing habits in multiple reports. Monitoring is clearly important, but our decisions sur-rounding the medicines that we prescribe should not just be based on cutting costs. The key goal of all our decisions is to enable good health and functionality in our patients. Our endgame is about making and keeping people well. If we lose sight of that, it is at our peril. Unfortunately, the MMT has not only lost sight of it – it has completely left their radar screen.

As Karen's symptoms failed to resolve, her mood started dropping. Her ability to function became more and more restricted. She turned from a successful woman, earning good money, paying taxes, support-ing a happy, functioning relationship and considering starting a family, to a withdrawn, tearful shadow of her former self. She was unable to work and lost her job, which meant she had to claim benefits. This further upset her, and she became so difficult to be around that her husband eventually left her.

The bright, breezy, confident beauty who had first walked into the surgery had become a bloated, pale invalid. She could not understand what had happened to her, and neither could I. This person who had once been a fully functioning, highly contributing member of society was now stuck in rounds of benefit assessments and barely able to leave her house. I was at a loss as to what could possibly be going on. Her thyroid blood readings were all over the place, and she had had several hospital admissions. She was deteriorating in front of me, and it seemed that there was nothing I could do to help her.

Then one day she was not using her crutches when she came in to see me. She was walking, and there was the hint of a flush in her cheeks. When I asked her what had happened, she told me she had started taking a different version of thyroxine. She was buying it – illegally – from a pharmacy in Boston, USA. It was the original form of thyroid replacement that had been used in the mid-to-late twentieth century, and was called Armour Thyroid.

I had never heard of it, so I did some research. I found out it was a prescriptible medicine in the UK, but was hardly ever used anymore. It was more expensive than levothyroxine as it was still made from desiccated pig thyroid gland. The key difference, however, was that it contained not just T4, but also the active T3 component of thyroxine. As I read around the subject, I discovered an increasing school of thought among endocrinologists that some people's bodies were simply not able to convert T4 to T3. For them, prescribing T4 alone was useless.

Over the next few months, Karen's life turned around. She stopped using her crutches entirely and returned to work. Her bounce and vitality returned and she presented a prestigious charity award. She was back in the game.

Early on in her recovery, I agreed to take over the prescribing and monitoring of her Armour Thyroid. It was clearly hugely beneficial to her. There were some slight increased risks, as the T3 level is higher in pigs than in humans, but after careful counselling and deliberation, we decided that the risks were far outweighed by the benefits to her overall health and wellbeing. Prescribing Armour Thyroid to Karen made sense on a health economics level, too. Although the medication was more expensive, and this increased cost was being borne by the taxpayer, the reduction in Karen's hospital bills more than made up for the this. Karen was once again an active contributor to the public purse through her taxes, and no longer claiming disability benefit. It was a win-win situation – or so I thought.

Then one day I got a call from the MMT which led to my first meeting with Rachel, our local MMT pharmacy representative.

Rachel was a pharmacist before joining the MMT; she no longer saw patients and spent most of her time reviewing data on large spreadsheets, to assess trends in prescribing and look for potential savings. Much of her work revolved around switching the NHS contracts from one brand of medicine to another.

Rachel was not happy that I was prescribing Armour Thyroid to Karen. Levothyroxine costs about £27 per month whereas Armour Thyroid is more like £270. She came to the practice to discuss it.

We sat in one of the small rooms upstairs. There were a few other nurses and doctors present, and Rachel looked uneasy. She was a small lady with grey skin and a permanent furrow in her brow. Her hair was drawn back and clamped into a ponytail, but wisps escaped around her face. She made small, staccato blinks of her eyelids when she talked.

'There is no evidence that Armour Thyroid works any better than levothyroxine,' she said to me. 'All the trials show no statistical difference. It is not cost effective.'

'Trials show that 98 per cent of people can't tell the difference. That means that 2 per cent of people can,' I replied.

'That is not significant. There is no evidence for its use. Our lead GP in the MMT says there is no evidence, and all the local endocrinologists agree.' I was sure I heard some triumph in her voice.

'Well – there is evidence,' I explained. 'There is the patient's evidence. There is the evidence of Karen's experience. Armour Thyroid has transformed her life.'

'N=1, Laura, N=1.' Rachel almost spat the words back at me.

She meant that Karen's positive experience – the total transformation of her life – was considered a trial of 1. Karen could be dismissed as an irrelevance, a number so small that it has no value.

I remembered my days as a medical student, when evidence-based medicine – or EBM as it became known – was just coming into being. It was a revolution. Giant pharmaceutical companies erupted into the world. They commanded mega budgets, which could fund hugely expensive trials, where N=20,000 or more. They sponsored meetings, educational events, dinners, hospital wings and equipment. Everything I owned at that time, from my pens to my books, tendon hammer and even paperweights, were branded by Bayer, Zeneca or GlaxoSmithKline. Big Pharma, big trials and big data ruled.

As doctors, we loved it. It appealed to our quest for scientific truth. We wanted to be 'sure' of the treatments we were using. The problem was that we became so enamoured of the 'sureness' of the data that we'd stopped believing our patients.

But I believed Karen. Her body did not respond to T4 – even if most patients' bodies did. Should I stop prescribing a life-changing medication that had a profoundly positive effect on her health? It had also significantly reduced the financial burden of her healthcare on the taxpayer – and surely, I thought, this was something that Rachel and I both wanted?

I asked her the all-important question. 'Is this my decision or yours?'

'Well, it's yours,' she replied.

Of course, it was mine. As Karen was my patient, I held clinical responsibility for her. I did not stop prescribing Armour Thyroid. The MMT continued to grumble at me in flurries of correspondence, but Karen's transformation was so clear that in the end, the argument ground to a halt. However, I didn't believe for one moment that the problem was solved.

N=1 was going to be a battleground. This had only been the first skirmish.

CHAPTER 4

Quality

In December 2014, the practice won a national award. We were named as Innovators of the Year at the National GP Awards Ceremony. The night we collected our award was amazing – one of the best occasions of my life. We'd been recognised as real pioneers. After all our hard work, we felt that we were really on the map.

My only real sadness on that wonderful evening was that Julie, my first inspiration, wasn't there to see it. Just before she died, I had told her of our plans to start a charity to fund the non-NHS services for people on low incomes. It was very important to us that these treatments, which had the potential to benefit everyone, were not limited to those who could afford them. The patients who could pay would do so, of course, and a percentage of their fees would go into the charity to help others. Julie heartily approved – she was an old lefty at heart.

We called it the Robin Hood Health Foundation. Our foundation has raised just under a million pounds over the last six years, and helped tens of thousands of patients to combine complementary therapies and arts programmes with their usual GP care. In the days that followed our awards success, I felt as though as I was walking on air.

But not long afterwards I fell back down to earth with a bump. We were facing our first CQC inspection.

The Clinical Quality Commission regulates and inspects health and social care organisations. It is the medical equivalent of Ofsted, the organisation that sends inspectors into schools. Sadly, its processes are just as punitive and stress-inducing. CQC's powers are wide and deep. It can shut a practice or a hospital down if they deem it unfit. A CQC inspection is a *very* big deal.

We had two weeks to prepare the practice for the visiting inspectors. The CQC website stipulates a long list of policies and protocols that are expected to be updated and in evidence at the practice. It threw us all into a high state of anxiety.

I spent a whole weekend writing policies on fridge temperatures, policies on kitchen-equipment storage, policies on what to do in the event of my death, policies on what to do in the event of anyone else's death, policies on our attitude to policies. (The policy on our attitude to policies is as follows: while a policy may be helpful in some situations, it is our policy not to blindly follow policy in case the blind following of policy prevents us from intelligently engaging with the situation that it was our policy to clarify – hence undermining the intention of the policy.)

Although we tried to face the situation with humour, we were all aware that the previous year CQC had shut down a practice next to us for not having the right policies. Nine thousand patients had to be reallocated and thirty people lost their jobs. All of the stress around the inspection gets layered on top of the ever-present anxieties that surround being at the forefront of primary care in the UK

The pressure gets to many people. Shortly before the inspection I heard that a GP and a GP trainee had both committed suicide. Four other local practices had to close due to difficulty in recruiting doctors. For some professionals, staying in the NHS no longer seemed worth the pressure: I had three friends and colleagues who were now sending images of happy, smiling, bronzed faces living a less stressful life in Australia.

As inspection day drew nearer, Gary couldn't sleep for three nights. He delivered a constant running commentary on what was happening, what everyone was doing and what they needed to be doing shortly.

Every time he talked about 'the choreography of the day', the assistant manager and secretary did a little dance routine behind him. It was one way to relieve the mounting stress we all felt. I was nervous too, but I had confidence in us. I was proud of every one of my team. All that was left was to show CQC what we were really made of.

With days left to go, CQC preparations rose to a peak of furious intensity. All the nurses were frantically cleaning and spraying and pulling out old bandaging and searching for imaginary dead rats behind the cupboards.

'What shall we do with Dr Hilary's old pictures?' asked Lara. She had found a new gear – MANIC HIGH – and was moving around the building so fast she had become a blue blur that was difficult to positively identify.

'Burn them,' replied Gary, without a moment's hesitation.

Two days prior to the inspection, on a Saturday morning, we cancelled all our patients' appointments. *Never mind about them – we have got to get this place ready or we'll get closed down,* was the overriding feeling.

It occurred to me that one of the categories we would be judged on was 'Caring'.

We were all working furiously when a patient arrived at the front door. She obviously didn't get the cancellation message. We could all see her through the large glass panel. Unfortunately, she looked unwell. The patient, Janet, was a lifetime smoker with severe lung disease. She was clearly in the throes of a terrible exacerbation, breathing rapidly through pursed lips and unable to talk in sentences. Her skin was blue.

'Don't let her in!' barked Gary, normally such a kind and gentle man. We didn't have time for patients. But Janet was so clearly struggling that in the end, we had to turn the locks and admit her.

'Okay – but don't give her any oxygen. We won't be able to replace it by Monday. That means instant closure.'

Janet's oxygen saturation levels had other ideas; they were right down, even by her usual standards. She was very poorly and needed low-level oxygen and nebulisers, which we brought her in to administer while we waited for the ambulance. As her lungs expanded and her brain was reoxygenated, she began to pick up. She wished us 'Good luck' as she was carted off by the paramedics.

It was not until after they were gone that we realised they had taken our whole oxygen canister with them. Now, not only did we not have any oxygen – we didn't even have a canister. There was a clear gap over the OXYGEN sign in the nurses' room.

This was the moment when I thought Gary might just walk out of the building. Emigrating to Australia seemed a real and viable opportunity.

We phoned the Royal Sussex Hospital, but they couldn't lend us a canister. It was late on a wintry Saturday afternoon by now, and growing dark. None of the other practices in our neighbourhood would open until Monday morning.

In the end we were saved by Sue, who called in a favour. The plan was that she would go to her mate's practice at 8 a.m. on Monday, as soon as they opened, 'borrow' their oxygen, then get back here for 8.30 a.m. We would meet the inspectors and take them to the Fire Assembly Point, which was mercifully at the back of the building, and talk to them there until we got the all-clear that Sue had managed to sneak into the front door and replace the oxygen canister. What could possibly go wrong?

By midnight on Sunday, the practice was shining, and the staff were scrubbed and clean with short nails, washed hair and caring smiles. Gary and I came in at 6.30 a.m. on Monday. I was in my suit. We had constructed a thirty-minute PowerPoint presentation outlining the progress we'd made with this once 'struggling practice'. In the time we had been here, we would proudly explain, we had turned it around. We'd won national awards and been recognised as a beacon of hope – a ground-breaking operation. I opened my laptop and placed it on the meeting-room table, ready for my grand presentation. Then I stepped outside into the hall and gave my waiting team a confident smile.

This was it. I wished I could shake the feeling that everything I'd fought for was on the line.

*

I first met Delilah just after her fifth husband had died. She looked about seventy-five but was, in fact, almost ninety years old. She was wonderfully frank about the enormous amount of plastic surgery she'd had, which had left her with a slightly odd appearance. One of her plastic surgeons had become her third husband.

Over the years she had amassed considerable wealth. She lived in a large Regency house on one of the squares by the sea. She was a lady who lunched – a lot. She periodically came to see me with aches and pains, and sometimes to ask me to sign her off as fit for her latest operation. 'This one's just a little tuck, darling,' she would say to me with a mischievous wink. 'Beautiful surgeon… ' She was always immaculately dressed with coral-pink nails, and 'ice' that would rival that of the most ostentatious of rappers.

After the death of her fifth husband, things started to unravel slightly for Delilah. She grew a bit too fond of her crystal sherry decanter, and this, combined with a low-level diazepam addiction she had picked up in the Eighties, made her increasingly unsteady on her feet. She tottered down to the shops and was frequently escorted back by paramedics or a handsome passer-by. Either scenario suited Delilah just fine. She was very persuasive when it came to luring her rescuers into her sherry-decanter lair.

Delilah would not go out without her make-up and jewels, and this made her incredibly vulnerable. After a particularly bad fall, which threatened to mis-shape her expensive nose, she took to drinking alone or on the phone to someone. Pretty much anyone would do. As many of her *bon vivant* companions had long since left this earth, she became a fairly frequent caller to the practice. The receptionists would chat to her, while remaining mindful of the host of other patients trying to get through. We referred her to a befriending service – a wonderful project that arranges for vetted volunteers to visit housebound patients in their homes and have a cup of tea or read to them, or help with shopping or things around the house. Delilah loved it and soon had far more volunteers than one person was permitted.

Gradually, though, her drinking had increased. She reached the stage where half of her waking life was spent trying to work out what had happened during the other half. She had more frequent falls. Neighbours worried about her and called the paramedics, but she refused to go back to A & E again after they offered her undrinkable tea and left her on a trolley in a hospital corridor for eight hours. She'd rather die, she said, and I think she really meant it.

One day I was called out to see her by a neighbour who had heard shouting. I tried to open the front door with the spare key from outside, but there was something blocking the door on the other side. I managed to open it a tiny crack and a diamond encrusted finger shot out of the gap at floor level. With some encouragement and direction, Delilah managed to roll away from the door she was blocking, and I was able to squeeze in and try to pick her up. She wasn't sure how long she had been there, but it couldn't have been long. Her knee was bruised, and a skin flap had come off her forearm. There was a small bump on her head.

She was shaken but quite quickly recovered her poise. We bandaged up her arm and she had a cup of tea. I'm pretty sure she would have had a sherry if I hadn't been there. I asked for her help in trying piece together the sequence of events of the preceding few hours.

She took to this exercise with alacrity, and some obvious experience.

'Well,' she said, 'I remember having dinner with Lucas.' (Lucas was the cat.) 'We had better go downstairs and see what happened down there!' She turned excitedly. 'There may be more clues!'

I followed her, a slightly unwilling Watson behind a deranged Holmes. I really should have had a notebook.

We went down the stairs. 'Aha!' she exclaimed. 'That needs analysis!' She pointed at a very large pool of dark liquid under the kitchen table.

'Could be red wine or... ' she paused for effect '... it could be blood!'

There certainly was, in my view, equal probability of either being true. On closer inspection I was able to pronounce it 'Red wine!'

We went back to our investigations. There was a plate on the table with some half-eaten food. There was a wine glass, which still had some wine in it. We moved on. It appeared, from the splatters of blood and some smashed cups, as though someone in the not-too-distant past had head-butted the Welsh dresser with some force. This could explain the bump on her head, I suggested to her.

'Yes, yes!' she interjected enthusiastically. 'I think we are getting there.'

She almost tripped again on a large rug at the top of the stairs as we climbed back to the living room. We went to sit on the sofa, dangerously close to the sherry decanter. Her eyes flicked towards it. Lucas shot off as we approached, clearly unnerved by the kamikaze antics of his mistress.

'Delilah,' I said, 'I am a bit worried that you might not be very safe here anymore.'

'Nonsense, don't overreact! You doctors are always overreacting. Bernie was like that – that's why I left him. He'd turned into a terrible bore.' She waved her hand, dismissing boring Bernard.

I tried another tack. 'Would you like some more help in the house? With cleaning and stuff?'

'Oh, maybe,' she replied, deflated. 'Ask Poppy. She will sort it out.'

'Okay, but please be careful, Delilah,' I said as we parted. I did realise that this was a pretty feeble statement, rather like shouting 'Watch out!' to young children as they scale a precipice.

Later I had a long chat with Poppy, Delilah's daughter, who was at her wits' end. She had been trying to persuade her mother to go into a nursing home. 'She won't go. She thinks she is Brigitte Bardot,' Poppy said. Apparently, Delilah was not willing to be around 'all those old people'. Getting carers in seemed the next best thing, along with a Carelink alarm for Delilah to wear around her neck. She wouldn't put it on. I couldn't help but wonder whether she might have been more willing if it had been diamond-encrusted.

My advanced nurse practitioner, Jacqui, went to check up on her a few months later. Nothing had changed. She found Delilah sitting in bed, bedecked in diamonds with a full face of make-up on and her hair done up. She was drinking rosé and talking to a double-glazing salesman on the phone.

We knew that she would probably fall over at some point and really injure herself, or even die… but I knew that was okay, because it's her life and she's living it just the way she wants. And until then, she will be Brigitte Bardot, almost ninety years old and still fabulous.

My vision of Delilah in her diamonds faded abruptly as the buzzer on the front door loudly sounded. The inspectors had arrived, with their clipboards and thin smiles. I smoothed down my jacket, cleared my throat and stepped forward to meet them.

*

The inspectors marched into our waiting room. We all stood together in a nervous little group. *So – first things first. Right now, that canister of oxygen is still missing. If that's spotted, it means an immediate fail.* As we began to show the group around, starting with a visit to the back of the building, I took a swift glance through the front window. To my massive relief, I saw Sue jumping out of her car with the bulky oxygen canister shoved up her jumper.

We're going to get away with it. We're good.

As part of the process, we introduced the inspectors to our patients. Helen and her daughter Jana were first. Jana was sixteen years old and the victim of online and school bullying. Born with a brain injury, she had restricted use of her left arm. After her father left the family home she began self-harming, making deep cuts to her arms and thighs and obsessing about her own death. She'd stopped going to school, and retreated into herself.

I'd referred her to CAMHS, the Child and Adolescent Mental Health Service, which had all but been disbanded. The reduction in mental health provision for the young is one of the greatest tragedies of the recent period of austerity. So much illness and crime are rooted in childhood trauma. And yet it remains the most underfunded and poorly staffed area of the NHS.

So CAMHS referred Jana to a charity called YAC, which stands for Youth Advice Centre. YAC provides short-term help to young people in crisis, but it does not have the skilled psychotherapists and psychiatrists required for a case like Jana's. YAC's inability to help her felt like another rejection to Jana. This is such a common story. So many vulnerable young people struggle to find appropriate mental health support.

That was why we had decided to provide this support ourselves. We employed our own art psychotherapist to run one-to-one sessions and groups for teenagers and young children with mental health issues.

Jana was one of them, and she turned out to be an incredible artist. She responded wonderfully to the help and support we gave her.

'It's really helped to see the art therapist,' she explained shyly. 'My mum – I think my mum was really worried. She wasn't sure how to help me. And I – I couldn't really explain – it was difficult. But when I started painting, everything got easier.'

The inspectors seemed happy. By early afternoon, I thought things were all going pretty well. The inspectors were impressed with our efforts to reduce the prescription of addictive drugs. Many of our addicts were in multiple crises, suffering with serious mental illness as well as substance misuse. Often, such patients are also homeless, having slipped out of the framework of society completely. They come through our doors addicted, traumatised, injured and in emotional and physical pain. They are some of the most fascinating and rewarding patients to treat – but keeping up with their often chaotic and dangerous lives can present significant challenges.

Next, the inspectors had a long talk with Shilpa the pharmacist. She was more than ready for them, her folders of protocols and research papers assuring them that all our prescribing and drug-monitoring protocols were in order. We expected that her rigorous checking and rechecking, along with her up-to-date knowledge and meticulous eye, would play right into their 'sweet spot'.

By 4 p.m., early winter darkness had fallen. One of the inspectors was murmuring something about 'a tight ship'. They were clearly impressed that we had managed to get a handle on the use of addictive medication. The ordeal must be nearly over. Everyone was starting to relax.

We gathered in the waiting room once more, preparing to say our goodbyes to the inspectors. The practice had been functioning as usual during the inspection and we paused momentarily to absorb the ongoing hum of activity around us. Then one of the consulting-room doors banged open – and out walked Ellen.

Every practice has an Ellen. Fifty-six years old, Ellen Shutters suffers with chronic and enduring anxiety, bordering on psychosis. She called the practice between twenty and fifty times a day, usually opening with the phrase: 'I am not well – I am really not well this time.' She often wanted a home visit and more medication – but she could generally be placated with a sandwich.

We'd taken steps to control the situation. Ellen had been banned from calling the paramedics and out-of-hours service, and even from calling Millview, the psychiatric unit. She was also banned from making 111 calls. But despite our best efforts to manage her condition, she was on enough medication to fell a small pony.

As she lurched out of Jacqui's door, she tripped on the completely smooth floor and banged into the radiator. 'I think I've broken my leg!' she screamed, staggering for effect and clutching the wall. We all stood there watching the scene, which looked like a horror movie in slow motion.

Jacqui rushed over to her. 'You're fine, Ellen – just a little bang.'

'No, I've broken my leg!' wailed Ellen. 'I've taken too much clonazepam again! I can't feel my feet! My head has gone numb! I think I might be dying!'

Her words seemed to echo down the corridor, then reverberate back, ringing round the ceiling, getting louder and louder.

Jacqui almost carried Ellen to the door, glancing nervously back at the inspectors. Once she had got to the porch, Ellen fell dramatically onto her mobility scooter. She weaved off into the night, dodging people and oncoming cars.

No one spoke for a few moments.

'Would you like a cup of tea?' one of our receptionists asked the inspectors. 'Or maybe something stronger?' she joked. 'Clonazepam, perhaps?' They didn't want anything and left immediately.

We made our way slowly back upstairs. Out of the topmost window, we could almost see our dreams of being awarded 'Outstanding' disappearing, veeringly wildly down the main road on a poorly driven mobility scooter.

For a moment, no one spoke. Then the team slowly dissipated around the building, absorbed back into our daily working rhythms. At 6.30 p.m., Jacqui posted a message on our internal messaging system. It was only one word long.

'Pub?'

There was a general consensus that this was an excellent idea. After the last patient had left, we locked up and made our way out of the building. As I closed the door behind us, I paused to look at the waiting room with its colourful paintings and lines of wishes still pinned on the wall.

The words: *I wish we get awarded 'Outstanding'* flashed into my head. But we wouldn't now, of course. Not after Ellen and her clonazepam. I just hoped they weren't going to fail us.

In reality, of course, it's impossible to measure the factors that are really important in medicine in an inspection. The difference you can make to someone's life and sense of wellbeing and health exists in another realm of language and communication, and is often not quantifiable in numbers or presentable in a graph. It can't be seen in a visit that lasts just a few hours. I could only hope that the inspectors had gained at least a sense of this while they were with us.

*

Three months, later the CQC's report and verdict were delivered back to us.

We received a grade of 'Outstanding Practice' in one area, but the rest were 'Good'. The inspectors had picked up that on two occasions over the course of the past three years the fridge temperature readings, which must be measured and noted twice a day at least, were missing.

We could have been deeply annoyed by this but, by that point, we had moved on from the inspection. We'd just been awarded a grant from the Arts Council to fund our Healing Arts Programme. The programme had started as a voluntary project run by artists and writers who gave as much time as they could to help patients express themselves creatively with paints or charcoal or modelling clay or words. This new funding had allowed us to hire a project manager, Emma – an author and literary scholar. Fiercely intelligent and passionate about her work and about her colleagues, she immediately set out to transform the volunteers' network into a vibrant organisation, which would go on to win recurrent funding.

Inspired by initiatives like this, we were able to laugh at Ellen's cameo appearance and the two missed recordings of the fridge temperature rather than dwell on the the fact that we hadn't quite achieved the grading we'd hoped for.

I went to speak to Lara, whose job it was to read and record the fridge temperature. I wanted to ensure she did not feel bad about what had happened.

'Darlin', darlin',' she replied in her strong Polish accent, 'fuck the fridge. There's more to life than fridges.'

For a moment, I wondered about making this the practice's strapline.

There were also some very proud moments as we read the CQC inspectors' report. They noted that 'this practice has an unusually warm and welcoming feeling'. And they 'had never inspected a place where there was such positivity and enthusiasm expressed so consistently by the staff about their workplace'.

We'd take that.

PART 2

Caring

CHAPTER 5

Fragmentation

There are some patients you just immediately love. For me, Darren was one of those patients. He reminded me of my son. Maybe I reminded him of his mum. He was a tall, good-looking seventeen-year-old boy. He had pale skin and wide eyes, and an endearing awkwardness that afflicts most boys his age. Every space he inhabited seemed too small for him, and uncomfortable.

Like many kids his age and many before them, he had been smoking a lot of weed. He and his friends appreciated the way it made everything funny and a little bit weird. Usually that hilarious, light weirdness wore off after an hour or so. Even when it wasn't that funny, and bordered on being uneasy and unnerving, Darren knew the feeling would soon subside and he would be back in the real world – though to be fair, the real world could also be unnerving and often downright distressing. He found something reassuring about the clarity of reality, even if the situation he was in in the real world wasn't ideal.

But recently, Darren had begun to notice that the weirdness he experienced while smoking weed was not vanishing once he was 'straight'. Voices and visions would come into his head and linger for days at a time. He had become paranoid about his friends. He was haunted by thoughts of self-harm that frightened him, even though he was able to dismiss them. He stopped going out after school. He wasn't sleeping. He stayed in his room. He smoked more weed to silence his now-actively psychotic mind. His behaviour scared his mum; an attractive blonde woman who worked hard to provide for her growing son.

There can be many different triggers to psychosis: dramatic life events, head injuries and drugs, for example. Many patients with mental illnesses who have access to psychotropic drugs, like weed, will use them to try to keep their symptoms at bay. That, I thought, must be what Darren was doing.

He sat in my consulting room looking at his hands, which were clasped on his knees. His low mood was palpable, filling the space. No matter how hard I tried, I couldn't get him to talk. Psychiatrists often say that you can tell how someone is feeling by how they make you feel. Angry, frustrated people will engender that feeling in you. Highly anxious people will make you also feel nervous and on edge. People suffering from depression can suck the life and colour out of a room. For this reason, they can be the most difficult patients to see.

For me, depression is the worst illness of all. We live in our heads, so our perception of the world is more important than how it actually is. Give me MS and a happy mind – but please, God, spare me the dark hopelessness of depression. Sitting with Darren, I felt extreme sadness radiating from him. But I didn't sense the devastating void or desperation of suicidal intention.

I tried to get him to open up about his mood and his feelings. But he was very hesitant and wouldn't really talk. He struggled to make eye contact and looked totally exhausted. We agreed he would try to stop smoking weed to help him sleep. He was willing, he said, to try a low-dose antidepressant medicine. I offered him group therapy, which he refused point-blank.

'Nah, doc. I can't handle that.'

'How about one-to-one counselling?' I suggested. 'Someone for you to talk to. They won't tell you what to do. They'll listen, and they might say something helpful.'

He didn't look too sure, but he eventually agreed. I knew I'd have to refer him to CAMHS as he was technically still a child, although I knew from experience, with patients such as Jana and many others, that they operate on about a tenth of the capacity required to provide this vital service to our most vulnerable children.

Darren needed to be seen urgently, and I was very worried that the system would respond too slowly. I suspected that CAMHS would reject my referral – and indeed that's what they did. Many times, in fact. Each time the referral was bounced back, weeks had passed by. And the longer Darren was stuck in his low mood, the harder it became to get him to believe that he would ever recover from it.

Finally he was given an appointment. But it was at a clinic that was a long way away from his home. By now he was too unwell to travel anywhere apart from the places he knew. He didn't attend the appointment, so he was discharged. I referred him again, explaining that I was worried about him. This time the letter I received suggested he would be better served by the Drug and Alcohol Team.

Darren was trapped. He needed to stop smoking weed before the Mental Health Team would assess him. But weed was the only thing that prevented distress and trauma taking over his mind. Without the softening, dulling effects of weed, he was terrified that his dark feelings might get out of control.

*

Julia had MS – a cruel, progressive form of the disease. It started with weakness in her right leg. Then she lost some sensation in her arm. Slowly, the disease took away the power and sensation in all her limbs.

For four years she used an electric chair but then her core became so weak that she had to have a large, fully supported, attendee-operated chair. But she couldn't spend more than a few hours sitting in it. Most of the time, she lay in a hospital bed on a mattress that undulated constantly, changing the contact on her skin so she did not develop pressure sores on a body she could neither feel nor move.

Julia used to be a dancer. She said she wasn't very good, but judging by the pictures on her walls, I thought she probably had been.

When I first met her, she had come to see me about her hip. Her lack of mobility had resulted in a tightening of the ligaments and the hip had become stuck in a bent position, as though frozen in a deep squat. Its position made changing her clothes difficult for Max, her carer.

Julia's speech was slow and drawling. Her articulation took effort and a high degree of concentration. She told me about Mr Erquay, an orthopaedic surgeon, who had offered to operate on her hip to free the contractures. She had been to see him five times, and each time the letter back from him read: 'We have decided not to operate for the moment but do refer Miss Bennett back if she would like to review this decision.'

I asked Julia what happened when she visited Mr Erquay.

'He just looks at the notes,' she says. 'I think there is something wrong with him, you know, up there.' She blinks her eye at me, and I get the impression that if she were able to move her arms she would be tapping her temple to indicate his gross stupidity. Perhaps unfairly, orthopaedic surgeons are not known for their emotional intelligence. I therefore referred her back to him again, spelling out the situation in as simple and clear terms as possible. But following the visit, yet another letter came back with the same final phrasing. 'We have decided not to operate for the moment but do refer Miss Bennett back if she would like to review the decision.'

'Right, that's it,' I declared to Julia. 'He is clearly a complete moron.' Julia slowly and deliberately nodded her head in agreement. I phoned Mr Erquay's secretary, and by some miracle learned that he was standing right beside her desk at that moment. The secretary passed him the receiver.

I prepared myself to issue a stern rebuke of his failure to take a proper history from this vulnerable patient.

'Mr Erquay, I am calling about Miss Julia Bennett, D.O.B 12.12.68,' I began.

'Oh yes,' he replied. 'She thinks you may have something wrong with you, you know, mentally. She can't understand why you keep referring her to me.' I could picture him gently tapping his forehead.

I looked over at Julia, who was smiling calmly and kindly at me. I remembered that sometimes MS can affect your memory.

'Right, well,' I said. 'Thank you for your time.'

Max was a twenty-four-hour carer. I thought he might have been a past lover of Julia's, though I never asked. He cared for her with incredible devotion and tenderness. He received a Carer's Allowance and she received Personal Independence Payments, which she gave to him. It wasn't very much, but somehow they made it work.

'We don't go out a lot,' Julia told me. They watched *Love Island* instead.

Julia couldn't swallow very well, so she needed to have thickened drinks, which tasted disgusting. She got pneumonia sometimes, when the lack of coordination of her palate meant she inhaled her drink by mistake. She was also prone to getting urine infections as she couldn't pass urine naturally and had an indwelling catheter. Her immune system was sluggish, so these infections made her very unwell very quickly. But she bore it all with good humour.

One January, Julia nearly died of a urosepsis. This started with a urine infection, which spread into her blood and set up a cascade of events that caused all her organs to go into shutdown. Luckily, Max, who slept in an adjacent room with the door open, heard her making an unusual noise. He called 999 and she was immediately taken to hospital, where she spent the best part of a month in the Intensive Care Unit. Without Max, she would certainly have died.

In March, Julia came to ask me to write her a supporting letter to the Benefits Agency. I think I must spend about four hours doing this for patients per week, and am sure that this time is not factored into the government's cost/gain calculations. But then, it is hard for me to see how the current benefit system can be anything other than a vastly expensive form of bureaucratic torture for the very ill. The cost of refusing and challenging people's disability claims must be astronomical. The vast majority of refused claims then go to tribunal and are upheld. The cost of the courts and assessors and adjudicators is significant. And there is the hidden cost of the doctors' time writing letters and supporting patients through these traumatic experiences – which in many cases throws people who were well on the road to recovery back many years. Sometimes it affects them to the point that they stay sick, caught in an endless cycle of proving their illness to officials.

Julia had been refused funding for twenty-four hours-a-day care and had been allocated only twelve hours of care a day. What she was supposed to do the other twelve hours was anyone's guess. It was, of course, absurd. Julia would die pretty quickly without someone on hand around the clock.

'Did they actually see you?' I asked. 'And examine you?'

'Yes,' she said. 'They told me I did not tick all the boxes.'

I looked at her in her wheelchair. Max, next to her, lifted her arm, which had become squashed between the wall and the side of the chair.

It was impossible to imagine what criteria for 'box ticking' her profound disability could not fulfil. I started typing an indignant letter listing her severe lack of function and total reliance on carers. I read it out as I was writing so that she could interject if she disagreed with anything. As I came to the end, I looked round at her, pleased with my forceful prose.

But Julia was crying. Her tears rolled down her face and into her mouth. Max tried to wipe them away.

'What is it, Julia?' I asked. 'I am sure it will be okay. They will agree to it in the end.'

'I'm sorry!' she cried. 'I just feel like such a burden. I'm so sorry. I'm so sorry. You shouldn't keep me alive.'

I moved my chair closer to her and stroked her hand. I could feel my throat constrict with anger and frustration. For a moment, I couldn't speak.

How can we punish her like this? I wondered. How can we make someone so brave and so vulnerable be so ashamed? It is wrong and it must change. She needs respect and trust – that's all. Would it really be so hard to achieve?

'Julia,' I said, when I could rely on my voice, 'the moment I hear from the Benefits Agency, I'll let you know.'

She nodded slowly. I sat at my desk feeling terrible as Max manoeuvred her wheelchair from the room.

Our current benefit system is inhuman and vastly expensive. In my opinion, it is sometimes verging on abusive. We need bureaucracy and administration – of course we do. But they are merely processes. Our higher ambitions should be fairness and compassion. I believe that the whole system needs careful, ethical re-thinking. As it slowly breaks apart, patients like Julia are denied their dignity as human beings.

*

The next time I saw young Darren, he came into my room in a state of high anxiety. This was quite unlike any of our previous consultations.

87

He seemed to have deteriorated strikingly. As he paced around the room I could feel his fear and uncertainty; there was an unpredictability about him. He was talking quickly.

'I haven't slept for a few days. Can't sleep.'

He stopped pacing and looked down at the yellow clinical bin in the corner.

He turned his head sideways to watch me carefully as he pointed to the bin.

'There's no one in there, is there?'

I shook my head. The bin is about two feet high and twenty centimetres wide.

He nodded.

'I know that. Of course there is no one in there. I am going mad. I need to sleep. I tried to score some weed last night, but I ended up in the police station. I just got out this morning. I don't know what to do.'

He rubbed his eyes and his face as he spoke as if trying to keep himself present in the room. He was very ill.

I tried to convey as much calmness and confidence as possible, in order to compensate for his agitation and reduce his neurosis It sort of worked. We talked about what he was thinking. He had a clear understanding that he was dipping in and out of reality. He still had insight. Above all, I suspected that he really needed to sleep.

I called MHURS (the Mental Health Urgent Response Service), bracing myself for a difficult call. But to my great surprise, the person on the end of the phone accepted my referral.

'Are you sure you are okay to take him?' I double-checked. 'He is seventeen years old?'

'Yes, that is fine – but let me just make sure.' The MHURS clinician put me on hold for a few minutes and then came back on the line to confirm the plan of action. I would give Darren a tranquilising antipsychotic called quetiapine to take, and he would go home and try to sleep for a few hours before a member of the MHURS team could come out to assess him.

Darren agreed and we called his mum. She agreed to wait for him at home. She was desperate to get him help, as he'd become more and more distressed over the last few days. I gave Darren the prescription and he left the surgery.

Pretty soon, I would wish I had not let him go.

My afternoon surgery started, and I saw my first couple of patients uneventfully. At 3.30 p.m., I called Darren's mum between patients, just to make sure MHURS had got there okay.

She answered the phone choked with tears.

'We were waiting for the mental health people. He took that prescription that you got for him and he seemed to be okay – but then they rang up and said there was a problem.'

Immediately I had a sinking feeling.

'What kind of problem?'

'They said they couldn't see him 'cause he's only seventeen. They said it should be CAMHS, because he's a child. But I thought you said –'

She started crying even more.

'Anyway – he overheard all this, and – and – it was like he snapped.'

'Snapped how?'

'He started shouting that nobody cared – that we don't care, that the doctors don't care – saying that nobody will help him and he'll never get better.'

'Where is he now?'

'We don't know!' I could hear the rising panic in her voice. 'Then he shoved us out of the way and ran outside. We don't know where he is.'

I told her that I would call her back as quickly as I could, and that if Darren returned, she should call me. About an hour later, the phone rang. By now the situation had reached crisis point.

'He came back!' she said, very close to panic. 'God knows what happened. He's got a black eye and a huge rip in his shirt. There's blood on his head. And he's – he's breathing funny.'

'What do you mean – funny? Is he having difficulty breathing?'

'I think he's just really scared. He's kind of panting. We tried to calm him down but he won't listen.'

'Where is he now?'

'In his room.' Suddenly she burst into loud, frightened crying. 'Oh God! What's going to happen to him?'

'He needs the paramedics,' I said. 'He needs assessment of his head injury and urgent assessment of his mental health in a safe environment. They will need to take him to A & E.' His mum agreed, and I called the ambulance service for them.

I saw a few more patients. Midway through my third consultation, a message flashed onto my screen that the paramedics were on the phone. As the patient stepped outside, I picked up the phone and spoke to a paramedic called Lucy.

'Dr Marshall-Andrews? Hi – I've assessed Darren now and the head injury looks pretty minor. He's acting aggressively, though – I think he'd picked a fight in the street and that's how he was hurt. It didn't amount to much.'

'Is he showing signs of psychosis?' I asked her.

'I wouldn't say so, no. He has odd thoughts, he says. It's scaring him and he's not making much sense some of the time. But he still has insight, so I don't think he's psychotic.'

'He's capable of making decisions?'

'Yes – I'd say he is. That's why he won't agree to go to A & E.'

'What reasons does he give?'

'Apparently the last time he went in, there were arguments. He's saying that they threatened him. I don't think he's helping himself, to be honest, but he's genuinely scared and he's very insistent. He doesn't want to go.'

'Have you tried to persuade him?'

'Yes – yes, I have.'

'Would you mind putting him on the line?'

In the background I could just make out Lucy's voice quietly asking Darren if he'd speak to me. Then I heard his laboured breathing.

'Darren?' I said gently. 'Hello – it's Dr Marshall-Andrews. I understand you've hurt your head.'

'Yes! But I won't go to hospital! If I go there, they'll beat me up!'

'Darren, if I give you a promise that you won't be beaten up, will you –'

Darren started yelling very loudly. I couldn't make out any words, but he was clearly terribly distressed. I realised that all I was doing was increasing his agitation.

Back on the phone to his mum, I explained that the best option was for him to be seen at home by either MHURS or CAMHS.

'Can you hold on there?' I asked her. 'I'm trying really hard to sort out help for you as quickly as I can. I understand your frustration and how worried you are. I'm sorry that it's taking so long.'

She quietly told me that she understood – but I couldn't shake the feeling that I was letting her down by not being able to find a way to access help for Darren.

'I'm phoning for help right now,' I told her. 'I'll be back to you as quickly as I can.'

As MHURS had directed us to CAMHS, I called them. I went through Darren's case history.

Then there was a pause on the end of the line.

'This definitely needs to go to MHURS,' the woman said. 'They should deal with patients over sixteen years old. You'd better call them back.'

I called MHURS back. I spoke to a man who assured me it was CAMHS who needed to see Darren. He checked with his supervisor once more. It was under CAMHS' remit, he confirmed.

I was starting to feel my own stress rising. I called CAMHS back. I could tell that the woman on the phone was starting to get annoyed. It was definitely MHURS staff who needed to go out there, she repeated. I asked to speak to her supervisor. There was no supervisor on duty, no psychiatrist I could speak to. Just her, the duty worker.

I was in the middle of my surgery. The patient counter in the corner of my screen already showed two patients waiting, their appointments now running late.

'He is very unwell. He really needs to be seen,' I implored her. 'Is there a psychiatrist with you?' She gave a dry little laugh at the very idea.

'If he is that unwell, he needs to go to A & E,' she said again.

'But he's refusing to go, and he has capacity to refuse.'

'You need to call the paramedics,' she advised.

'I have,' I insisted. 'And they have seen him and assessed him and they feel he needs help, but he won't go with them to A & E.'

There was silence down the line. The patient counter jumped up. Now there were four patients waiting.

'He's not safe,' I continued. 'He was beaten up when he left the house. He needs urgent assessment for his mental health. He has a head injury – he needs help.'

'Aha,' she pounced. 'If he has a head injury, he really needs to go to A & E.'

92

I took a deep breath.

'He won't go. The paramedics have assessed his physical injury as non-significant. He needs mental health support.'

Five patients were waiting now. My frustration and desperation were starting to get the better of me. I could feel my hands starting to clench.

'Look, can you at least –'

'We don't see seventeen-year-olds as emergencies,' the woman snapped, interrupting me. She was as powerless to change this situation as I seemed to be. It was defensiveness, I realised, that was making her voice curt and rigid. 'What do you expect me to – are you crying?'

I gave up and put the phone down.

Another two message boxes popped up on my screen. One of them read: 'The paramedics are on line four about Darren.' Meanwhile, the second one informed me: 'Your next patient is getting very angry. They have been waiting for over forty minutes.'

I picked up line four, and heard the voice of Lucy the paramedic. Her shift had finished but she had gone back to the house to check on Darren. She was really concerned. He was becoming more and more disturbed and his mother was becoming increasingly scared of him. She knew what it was like for them, she said. I sensed this whole situation mattered personally to her. She assured me she wouldn't leave the family. I advised giving Darren another quetiapine tablet.

'And we had better call the police,' I advised Lucy. 'Darren needs a psych assessment, but I just don't seem to be able to get one.'

'Don't worry,' she answered, 'we'll work it out between us. Call me back in twenty minutes.' She gave me her mobile number.

I wanted to hug her.

I got through a few patients and then called her back. The situation was worsening. Darren was getting more agitated and distressed. The police had arrived. They could not take him against his will from his home. Lucy and I racked our brains for another route for a psychiatric assessment. Eventually, a policewoman suggested that his mother make an allegation against Darren. That way, they could take him to the police station under arrest and get him assessed by their forensic psychiatrist there.

It was far from an ideal solution. We all felt that being arrested and taken by force to a police station, put in a cell and then seen by the forensic psychiatrist was likely to significantly worsen his mental state. But we could not leave him alone in the house. He was becoming a risk to himself and to his mother.

I felt a physical pain at the thought of this child being handcuffed and taken to a police cell. And just as I had feared, it proved to be deeply traumatic. He completely lost touch with reality. Once in a cell, his paranoia became violent and his crisis escalated.

None of this should have happened. If the support services worked as they should do, professional help could have been provided for Darren when he first needed it. The longer he was left without support, the more acute his crisis was becoming. It's hard to watch fractured services losing people's lives down their gaping cracks. It is still incredible to me that there is this loophole in mental health provision for sixteen- to eighteen-year-olds.

During my training, one of my professors used to say to me: 'Medicine is easy, Laura, it's the patients who are difficult!' Nowadays a more fitting saying would be: 'Medicine is easy – it's the system that's difficult.' Finding a diagnosis is a whole lot simpler than trying to help patients through pathways of care that are all too often more like obstacle-filled assault courses. The only bright light in this dreadful situation was Lucy the paramedic, and her prompt and compassionate interventions. In situations where the system is fragmented and broken, sometimes people shine. In this case, she most certainly did.

I believe she saved Darren's life by going back after her shift and staying at the house. She saved his life not with her resuscitation skills or her sophisticated equipment – she saved him because she cared. She saved him with her ability to act beyond protocol, showing compassion for another person and acting on that feeling.

But I knew that a young man and his family were still at crisis point.

Two weeks later, I had a call from a psychiatrist in Liverpool.

'Liverpool?' I queried, though I really wasn't surprised. Darren had been transferred there from Brighton Police Station as it was the closest available bed for him – a distance of 270 miles. The consultant said that his was the most severe case of paranoid psychosis she had ever seen. He stayed there for three months. His mum travelled up and down to visit him as often as she could.

Maybe he would still have descended into florid psychosis if he had been assessed and treated at home – but maybe he wouldn't have. Who knows? It is impossible not to think that he was seriously let down by his health service at a time when he needed it most. As doctors, we are a team. Sadly, there is a big psychiatry-shaped hole in our team structure. All too often, when we turn to the psychiatrists in a moment of crisis, they are just not there. Instead, patients are left floundering in the dangerous waters of fragmented care.

Darren was discharged from his high-intensity, high-security treatment in the Liverpool unit. He is coping at the moment, but it's likely that he will start to flounder again. He has deeper issues that need addressing. But there is no funding for long-term therapy on the NHS anymore. Until we agree to prioritise mental health and dealing with the trauma experienced by children, patients like Darren will bounce, at vast expense to us all, in and out of psychiatric units.

CHAPTER 6

Pain

'The placebo effect is one of the most fascinating things in the whole of medicine. It's not just about taking a pill, and your performance and your pain getting better. It's about our beliefs and expectations. It's about the cultural meaning of a treatment.'

— BEN GOLDACRE

I was in my consulting room, about to begin my afternoon surgery. My first patient was Troy. This was not a good start.

I usually booked in Troy at the end of a surgery. Troy could not be rushed. He had his own agenda. Born in East London, he'd spent a year of his early life in Jamaica, but something difficult had happened there when he was very small, and his mother had picked up her five children and carted them back to an East London estate.

Troy was the youngest child, and his mother made no bones about the fact that she would much rather have had four. She was cruel to him, possibly embittered by his father's abandonment of her and the hardness of life as a single mother with very little money. She would shut Troy in a cupboard when he annoyed her, which was often. His siblings also blamed him for the family's misfortunes. He left home as soon as he could and disappeared into the shadowy margins of society.

Once he was on his own, Troy discovered that his sexuality and beauty could command a price, and he used them both. He hinted darkly at past misdemeanours with politicians and well-known businessmen. I guessed a mosaic of truth and untruth existed in his cloudy recollection. He had eventually left London and come to Brighton with a boyfriend who'd abandoned him too. Now he lived in a small council flat, unable to hold down a job or relationship and deeply suspicious of the world. He had picked up a plethora of diagnoses on his journey through life and now, at forty-six, he suffered from fibromyalgia, chronic fatigue, anxiety, schizoaffective disorder, oppositional and defiant personality disorder, and sometimes suicidal depression.

Such a long list was very discouraging. My GP trainer used to say that some patients would accrue as many diagnoses as psychiatrists they saw, as each would find a slightly different analytical perspective on the person's thoughts and behaviours. This was certainly the case with Troy. There was no clear consensus on what sort of mental illness he was suffering from, if indeed he was suffering from any mental illness at all.

I got up and walked out into the waiting room to call his name.

'Troy. Hi, Troy, come on in.'

He was an unmistakable figure, tall and slender with fine features, a high brow and hazel eyes that shone out brightly against his pale brown skin. He had once been a very handsome man, but now his looks had been ravaged by the harshness of his life. His teeth were yellowed and uneven and he had light stubble over his lower face. There were deep furrows in his forehead and a scar that ran down from his temple for about an inch, narrowly missing his left eye. He was sitting in the corner of the room, alert, watching the comings and goings of the practice intently.

Just as I had feared, he began our consultation with an attempt to confront me.

'Do you monitor your staff?' he asked as he sat down.

This felt like a dangerous question – a set-up.

'What do you mean?' I replied.

'Well – they seem to spend a lot of time walking around and chatting when there are patients waiting.' He looked at me intently, waiting for some sort of response.

I let it slide. I had fallen into these little barbed traps before. I wouldn't be derailed so early on in the consultation.

'How can I help you, Troy?' I smiled and gestured to the chair. It was cold outside and he was wearing a thick coat with a woolly hat pulled down over his dark curly hair. He remained standing as he slowly unwound the long green scarf from his neck and hung it over the back of the chair. He paused and then unbuttoned his coat, paying close attention to each button. He carefully smoothed the dark brown woollen coat and folded it over the chair as well. Then he removed his hat and stood for a moment wondering where to put it. He opted for the foot of the couch. He sat down, settling in, making himself comfortable.

'So, do you?' he said.

'Do I what?' I replied

'Do you monitor your staff?'

I sighed. 'Troy, could we focus on you?'

'Well, I think it's important that taxpayers' money is spent wisely.' He smiled in an oily kind of way.

'Thank you, Troy, I will raise your concerns with Maureen.'

'I'm just trying to help,' he explained, noting the edge in my voice.

'So – how are you?' I tried again.

'Not good.' With that, he was off on a familiar routine. He was in constant all-over body pain. He couldn't sleep and the pain was making him suicidal. If I couldn't give him something for the pain, he would surely kill himself. I had to fix it.

Troy felt this pain primarily in his back and pelvis, but despite extensive imaging and investigations, we had never been able to locate its physical origin. He was on a lot of medication already, and every referral I made for him layered another one on the top: the pain clinic had added gabapentin, the psychiatrist duloxetine, the back clinic amitriptyline... and so it went on. He claimed that nothing worked except morphine. At some point in the distant past, he had been started on long-acting morphine and quickly his dose had escalated. The thing about morphine is that you get used to it after a while. So you want more. I needed to bring the dose down; he wanted to increase it. The difficulty for me was that I didn't really have anything else to offer him. He had tried pretty much every medication I could think of. Everything else I suggested, he would reject. This was a ritual dance we did with too many patients who had slipped into opiate addiction.

After about fifteen minutes, he changed tack. He told me about a doctor who had been struck off for not prescribing adequate pain killers for her patient who then committed suicide, citing her in his suicide note. Then he moved on to the terrible situation he was currently facing with his neighbours and an ongoing feud. He felt persecuted and watched; it was playing into his paranoia. He was feeling suicidal. Underneath it all was the tacit implication that somehow this was all my fault. It was my inability to cure him that was to blame for his predicament. Any other doctor, he suggested, would be able to help him. I stood my ground.

'Troy, I really can't give you any more morphine. We need to reduce your dose, not increase it.'

'So what am I going to do for my pain? If you're not careful, you're going to have a dead body on your hands. My mate Phil said he is worried he's gonna come round to see me and find my body hanging from the ceiling. I'll do it, you know. I really will. I can't go on like this – it's intolerable. This is no life.'

His voice was rising.

'I'm sorry, Troy. We have to find something else.'

He started to shout.

'Well – what? What? I've tried everything, you've said that yourself. What are you going to do?' He was perched forward in his chair, leaning towards me to hammer the point home.

'What about acupuncture?' I suggested. 'Or osteopathy? Right here in this practice, we have –'

'Are you fucking kidding me? You're a joke! I can't take this anymore.'

He got up and marched to the door, peering outside to check there were at least a few people in the waiting room. Today he was in luck – it was full. He had an audience. He walked back to my desk, grabbed his coat and hat and scarf and stormed out, shouting as he did so:

'I am going to kill myself! No one will help me! It's all *her* fault!' I heard the front door slamming shut behind him.

I sat with my head in my hands for a moment, breathing deeply. Troy would be back. He'd write me a card apologising for his behaviour, and round we'd go again. His words, though, stayed with me through the rest of my surgery. I didn't think he would kill himself. But he was an impulsive male in his mid-forties with a strong history of trauma and neglect, and that was a high-risk demographic for serious self-harm. I had to take the possibility seriously.

His main focus was his physical pain. But I suspected that what he was feeling was related to the stored, unreleased pain of years of abuse and emotional scarring, which he was too defended and confrontational to discuss, finding expression through his body. I remembered Sarah, sitting calmly in the waiting room after she'd had a few sessions of acupuncture with Ben. Troy had rejected the suggestion out of hand, but I wondered if this treatment might help him start to make a connection between the symptoms in his body and his deep emotional state. I even thought, very briefly, of bribing him to give acupuncture a try – but that would never work and was ethically highly questionable.

I decided to try a direct approach instead and phone him. I'd never done this out of the blue before: we usually spent our time trying to avoid contact with Troy, rather than court it. My last patient left and I picked up the receiver and dialled his number. He answered.

'Hi, Troy, it's Laura, Dr Marshall-Andrews. I have been thinking about your pain.'

Silence.

'I really think acupuncture might help you. I'm not going to take your morphine away – but can we just try it? It's not available on the NHS, but the practice will fund it for you.'

He seemed taken aback that I had called him like this. He was off guard and therefore more open. There was another long pause.

'I thought you were calling to strike me off the practice.'

His voice was unsteady and quieter than usual. Then he was silent again. I wondered if he was still there, but I waited.

'All right,' he said. 'I'll try it.'

'That's great Troy, the acupuncturist will call you to arrange an appointment.'

*

Brian and John lived together in a small house near the railway. Brian had been a glorious actor who had strutted the boards in the West End of London and on Broadway in the 1960s and 70s. John had done some writing, but his life mainly revolved around the flamboyant Brian.

Now in their early seventies, they had fallen on harder times. I had been called out by John to visit Brian who was 'not doing well'. It was late in the afternoon when I arrived and knocked at their unkempt door.

Their house felt like a bony, skeletal figure hugging its thin shawl around it. Some houses give a sense of foreboding as soon as you walk into them – this was one of them. One felt as though there may be hidden horrors behind the doors. Gruesome Dickensian figures of neglected humanity came into my mind. It was cold and dimly lit. The entrance hall was narrow. I think the walls might once have been cream but it was hard to tell. A bare bulb hung over a solitary picture, which always hung at the same wonky angle, limply clinging onto the nail. It was a 1920s ink caricature of a young man with his bottom showing. John led me up the stairs. Bare, un-sanded floorboards were sparsely covered with threadbare rugs whose patterns had long since disappeared.

We arrived in the main upstairs room, which looked out over the road to the station. This was obviously the room they lived in. There was a small wooden table with two chairs beside it and a plastic bottle of R. White's lemonade standing on it. There was a small three-bar electric heater in the middle of the room, which had a dark, fraying lead extending to a black Bakelite plug in the wall. There was a single mattress on the floor, which was covered in a pale pink blanket. Under the blanket lay a man. Brian.

My first thought was that he was dead. As we approached, however, his right eye sprang open, and then his left eye too. He threw out his arms from under the covers and cried with extraordinary vocal projection, 'Are you an angel? Have I died?'

I looked back at John who went over to the table and sat down.

I knelt down next to Brian, who took my hand in his and implored me to 'make it quick' before turning his head on the pillow in a gesture of resignation.

I tried to ascertain the exact nature of Brian's symptoms. It was hard to pin him down on the details. Did he have a cough? Did he have pain? I examined him and he appeared to be in good health. His temperature was normal, his blood pressure was good, his pulse was strong and regular. His chest was clear, his abdomen was soft with no masses or tenderness. His muscular power was good and his reflexes normal. He was a puzzle. Apart from the fact that he thought he was dying, he seemed in excellent health.

I drew a number of vials of blood from the vein in his right arm, then knelt back and looked at him for a minute.

He turned his head and stared back at me. Tears oozed from his eyes and trickled onto the pillow.

'What can be done?' he asked, forlornly.

'I think you are actually quite well, Brian,' I replied. 'I can't find anything obvious wrong with you at the moment. We will see what the blood tests show. In the meantime, try to get up and have some supper.'

'They don't know what the matter is! John, do you hear that? There is nothing they can do.'

John didn't say anything. He got up from his chair and walked me back down the stairs, past the doors and the lopsided picture.

I was pleased to get out into the grey drizzle of Monday afternoon, with its bustle of ordinary life.

A few days later, Brian's extensive panel of blood results came back. They were all completely normal. His viral screen was negative, his markers of infection and inflammation were normal, his kidneys and liver were functioning fine, his bone marrow was working normally. His urine culture came back negative.

I went back to see Brian to tell him the good news. He looked thinner. John said he had stopped eating and was only getting up to go to the toilet. After much persuasion, we got him to go to the hospital in an ambulance to have a chest X-ray and heart monitoring. He was sent back – it was all normal. I wondered if he was depressed. He refused antidepressants, and the elderly-care psychiatrist pronounced him of sound mind.

A few weeks later, I went back to see him again. He was still lying under his pink blanket on his mattress on the floor. John put some rich tea biscuits on a small plate and offered me one. I politely declined. Brian was definitely losing weight. The muscle bulk in his legs was significantly less, and he was starting to develop red patches on his buttocks where the constant pressure of lying down was damaging the skin.

'Brian,' I said to him, 'you have to get up more. You will be fine. I can't find anything wrong with you.'

We tried to stand him up and he tottered weakly to the toilet and back before collapsing into his makeshift bed.

'Darling, it's over. I have had the most wonderful life. Haven't I, John, haven't I?'

John nodded over his rich tea biscuit. 'Wonderful.'

'Brian,' I said, 'you can still have a wonderful life. You are okay. Really, you are.'

'Do you really think so?' he replied. 'Really?'

'Yes.' I was emphatic. 'Yes, you are okay, I promise.'

Despite my promise, he died a couple of weeks later.

I didn't know what to write on the death certificate, so he had to have a post-mortem. No disease was found. Frailty of old age was the formal cause, but really I think deep down that he wanted to die and he'd created a fixed belief that he *would* die. He had had enough, and it was time to go. This belief was so powerful that it affected his body, to the point where it stopped working at all.

*

We are not even close to understanding the full extent to which our minds can control and influence our bodies. I think this will require a deep shift in our biomedical modelling of the human body.

But there is one thing I am sure of: that the way we perceive pain isn't the same for everyone. It is a personal thing, and sometimes very hard to predict. There is still so much that we don't understand in medicine.

If we stand on a nail, for example, sensory neurons fire messages, which often cause an involuntary contraction of muscles to remove the foot from the nail. These messages carry on up the spine to the brain, informing it of the event. Often at this point we feel a sensation in the foot, but the signal is not interpreted as pain. It's not until we look down and see the blood or the offending nail that we realise 'this hurts'.

There are many tribes and groups all over the world whose people can reach a meditative state in which they control these signals completely, and do not feel pain – like Sufists, who can walk on hot coals, or Hindu devotees who are able to suspend themselves from hooks pierced through back muscles, apparently without feeling any discomfort. Somehow, they can train their minds to filter out signals that would leave others screaming in agony. And even without mental training or spiritual ideas, the power of belief can have extraordinary effects. Dr Henry K. Beecher, an army medic treating casualties in Italy in the Second World War, was one of the first people to document the use of placebos in pain relief. During a particularly desperate period involving high levels of casualties, he ran out of morphine and was forced to operate on injured soldiers without giving them pain relief. Instead, he administered a saline solution, telling them it was morphine; 40 per cent of his cases reported they felt no pain at all, since they believed they would not.

But just as we can learn to filter out signals, we can also 'turn up' our awareness and heighten our sensitivity. For some people, fear and trauma can be locked into our neural system, emerging as pain.

*

Brad always brought me *Vanity Fair* magazines. He was not a tall man, but he had a big Australian presence. He talked loudly and with confidence about everything and anything. He often arrived at the surgery with a book. He loved intellectual tomes, which he would bang down on my desk with satisfaction. He would make casual reference to them during his consultation, as if the characters or events were all around us. He lived in a colourful world enhanced by his prodigious reading habit. He lived alone, but had a habit of meeting with a string of male companions who shared his love of saunas, from where he seemed to pick up syphilis with alarming regularity. Brad took this in his stride and would attend for regular penicillin injections whenever necessary.

Brad lived on almost nothing. He had inherited a small amount of money from an Australian relative some years ago, but had no other incomings. He had travelled frequently in the past but was now content to stay local, reading and walking up and down the seafront. He had a beautiful flat on the ground floor of one of the big Regency buildings on the seafront that was grand and eclectic, and that he loved.

His neighbour upstairs, Nancy, was the landlady and freeholder of the whole building. Brad checked on her daily and helped her with food and brandy shopping. In return, she gave him a significant reduction on his rent. It was a happy arrangement for them both.

Brad came to see me with low-level chronic pain in his right wrist. It was a constant ache that would not go. He used pot to self-medicate, which he swore was more effective than any medication he had ever been given by doctors. He also suffered from thinning of the bones from heavy-dosage HIV medication thirty years ago, and from arthritis in a number of his joints. He had had physiotherapy and osteopathy in the past, but nothing had really helped. He bore his pain, folded it up and carried it on his back like a light backpack that he barely noticed most of the time.

At one of our consultations, however, the pain had significantly worsened. Brad was clearly in agony. His speech was punctuated with grimaces and groans, and his left hand rubbed and squeezed his right wrist. The movement of his lower arm was restricted by the intensification of the pain. He had been smoking more pot and he was starting to cough, which caused spasms to tear across his body. He became tearful during the consultation. The discomfort he was in was unbearable, and to cap it all, Nancy was dying.

She had taken to her bed and was slipping in and out of consciousness. She had a nephew who was set to inherit her considerable estate, so not only was Brad losing a friend, he was also potentially losing his flat. Nancy did not really like her nephew. According to her, the young man was a shrew: narrow-minded and business-focused with no love or generosity of spirit or soul. He hated her brandy habit and the off-beat, tapestried disrepair she lived in.

In the past, Brad had been addicted to morphine. I was therefore loath to give him painkillers related to this powerful drug, and he was already taking a plethora of pain medication. We referred him for urgent imaging of his wrist to exclude cancers or other deep pathology. He had blood tests and urine tests and saw several different specialists. His arthritis was undoubtedly present, but his images were not significantly different to several years ago.

We spent months adjusting his medication and experimenting with different forms of therapy. His pain would not respond. It kept him up at night and stopped him eating. He could no longer go out walking along the seafront. All he could do was sit with Nancy, comforting her in her last few weeks.

He still brought me recent copies of *Vanity Fair*. I offered him counselling and antidepressants, which can help with pain. We managed to get him to a pain clinic, and they tried some deep nerve blocks in his wrist and gave him a TENS machine, which treats pain by generating a mild electric current. It didn't help.

And then, one day, Brad walked into my room. He was standing differently, appeared taller and looked about ten years younger. He was holding *Bring Up the Bodies* by Hilary Mantel. He put the book down on my desk and lifted both his arms out on either side of his head like a runner crossing the finish line.

'It's gone!' he cried. 'I can't believe it, it's gone!'

'What did you do?' I asked, incredulously.

'Nothing!' he replied in equal amazement. 'Nothing!'

He sat down, moving his wrist around to demonstrate his new-found suppleness and ease of movement. His skin appeared better, he had energy in his body and his face was animated. I was looking at a different man.

I asked him about the flat and about Nancy.

'It's the funniest thing,' he replied. 'She died last week and her nephew came down to see me, and do you know – he was so kind. Not at all the person I was expecting. He said I can stay in the flat as long as I want, and he won't change the rent. The next day, my pain went. I have never felt like this. Ever. It's a miracle.' He looked up at the ceiling as if expecting something extraordinary to appear there.

Brad's wrist became a useful barometer of his mood. We noticed that when he was lonely or contracted another bout of syphilis, his wrist hurt more. When a family member died, he had another bad spell of pain. His was a stoic personality, typical of his age group, brought up in an era when men did not cry. It was almost as if he was unable to register emotional pain, and instead his distressed brain fixed on a physical interpretation that it understood.

In the end, however, his unusual pain perception probably contributed to his untimely death.

*

It was a Tuesday morning in January. I was on call for the practice. In our practice, anything urgent is dealt with by the on-call or 'duty' doctor. That doctor sits up in the admin room with the staff who take the incoming calls from patients requiring appointments or medication or advice.

I was ploughing through my list of calls. Zoe, a bright, intelligent receptionist, picked up a call. I was aware of her questioning a patient on the other end of the line while I wrote my notes. I turned to look at her, noticing that she seemed worried. GP's receptionists deal with hundreds of patients a day. They become pretty good at recognising symptoms and signs, so I took her concern seriously. She passed the telephone receiver to me. I checked her computer. Brad's notes were up on the screen.

'Hi, Brad?' I began.

'Hi, Laura,' he said in his unmistakable Australian drawl. 'I don't want to make a fuss, but I have this odd feeling in my stomach.' His voice sounded weaker than usual, and forced, as if speaking required a lot of effort.

'Yeah,' he continued. 'Few days now, I can't really do anything. Do you think I have food poisoning again? I had a Chinese... ' His voice trailed off.

I asked him if he had pain. 'Well, it's not as bad as my wrist was, but it doesn't feel normal,' he replied.

There was a long pause.

'Brad? Brad?' He took a few seconds to reply.

'Yeah?'

'Brad, is anybody with you?'

'No, no, I'm alone.'

'Brad, I am calling the paramedics. Can you get to the door? They won't be long.'

'No, don't do that, I'm not that bad. Sounds a bit overkill.'

'Brad, I'm going off the line now, but I will call you back in a minute.'

I called 999. I wasn't too sure what was going on with Brad, but sometimes heart attacks can present with abdominal pain. He didn't sound at all well in any event. The 999 operator answered quickly. After we had ascertained that my patient was not actively bleeding, had not sustained a head injury, lost consciousness or gone blue, a 'blue light' ambulance was dispatched.

I tried to call Brad back, but the line was engaged. I got on with my notes but kept my antennae out for the paramedics calling back.

Twenty-five minutes later, they called. Our receptionist, Zoe, passed them on to me.

'Hi – Dr Marshall-Andrews?' a young male voice came down the phone. 'We have arrived at the address. I'm afraid the patient was DOA. Sorry, it took us a while to gain entry. He still had the phone in his hand.'

DOA means dead on arrival. My brain froze and I couldn't think properly. 'What?' I whispered.

'Dead on arrival, doctor, sorry. We will notify the coroner.'

I put the phone down and stared at the computer screen. I picked up the phone and called my next patient. After a few patient calls, I stopped feeling sick. About an hour later, I had a message from Reception downstairs. The paramedics were at the desk asking for me.

I went down quickly. Sometimes an ambulance crew brings in patients who aren't ill enough to visit A & E, but who need to see a doctor.

A young paramedic was standing at the desk in his dark green uniform. He had short dark hair and a smooth, kind face. He exuded calm and confidence. I looked behind him for the patient. There was no one there.

'Hi, doc,' he said. 'We just thought we'd swing by and check on you. You sounded a bit upset on the phone. Did you know that chap well, who was found DOA? It took us about twelve minutes to get the door down. You did what you could.' He patted me a couple of times on the back.

'I'm fine,' I said. The young paramedic left, and I walked back through the waiting room to the toilet where I threw up.

Brad died of an ischaemic bowel. A blood clot had lodged in one of the arteries supplying his bowel which caused the muscle to die, rather like a heart attack of the bowel. A bowel attack. He must have had pretty bad pain for a few days, but he didn't register it as a threat.

It was extraordinary to think that Brad's mind could have been as powerful as this. Belief had controlled the signal his brain received, and the idea of 'food poisoning' had made his pain bearable. I was deeply sorry for his death, but at least, I thought, he hadn't been afraid. He never knew there was a problem at all.

*

Jasper and Jake lived together in a big modern apartment. It covered two floors, and sometimes their friend Wilbur lived there too. Jasper and Jake were heavily tattooed. At the weekends they wore DM boots and vests that exposed their inked bodies. In the week, they both worked in a bank and Wilbur worked on the railways.

Jasper and Jake had both contracted HIV in the late 1980s. Most of their friends died. They survived with a combination of gruesome drugs that suppressed the AIDS virus, but also destroyed much of the protein in their tissue, eating into the muscle bulk of the face, leaving them with well-defined ligaments in their cheeks and hands. This is the specific look of the survivors of early medications such as Atripla. Many of the difficulties faced by early survivors of HIV infection are still due to the damage wreaked in their bodies by the only treatments that were available at the time; brutal sledgehammers that were desperately fighting a terrifying foe.

Jasper was a long-term sufferer from chronic pain in his back and legs. He had osteoporosis (thinning of the bones), which was probably a consequence of his HIV treatment. His vertebrae had crumbled into each other and pressed on the roots of the nerves exiting the spinal cord and heading down the legs. Along with this, he had some difficulty in lifting his right foot. He found the pain he was in difficult to bear. It was likely, I thought, that this pain was associated with the deep trauma of living through the plague-like disease that devastated the gay community in the eighties and nineties. It was acting as a constant reminder of that horror.

Jasper was receiving therapy through one of the HIV charities. These charities are wealthy, well-funded institutions, which have made a great deal of research possible. For that reason, HIV is now one of the 'better' illnesses to get. Medications are much more sophisticated, and treatment is exceptional. The average life expectancy of sufferers approaches levels seen in the wider community. For those infected early on in the pandemic, however, it still remains a brutal disease.

Jasper was well known to the pain clinic. He'd been attending for years and, when I first met him, was on five different types of opiate medication: fast-acting forms, slow-acting forms, opiates combined with other medications, opiates in the form of patches and opiates in the form of lozenges. On each visit, another painkiller was added to his long list of medications. Opiates are medications derived from morphine. They are very effective painkillers, but highly addictive. In the past, they were used with alarming frequency, and the legacy of this practice is a generation of patients just like Troy and Jasper, who are addicted to these insidious drugs.

All these opiates often made Jasper confused and disorientated. Sometimes he would fall asleep in our consultation, mid-way through a conversation. On one occasion, he went into such a deep state of unconsciousness in the surgery that he had to be injected with an antidote and taken to hospital.

On one visit, he was suffering with the symptoms of a cough, and Jake thought he seemed confused. I was going to have to listen to his chest. This always required more concentration than a usual chest exam, because Jasper had explicit pornography tattooed over his back and chest. The images mainly consisted of large phalluses attached to various animals and each other. Maintaining a neutral expression during the examination required effort, especially if I noticed another graphic detail I had overlooked in previous inspections. Resisting the urge to gasp and look away was hard for someone brought up in a relatively sheltered environment. During this particular examination, Jasper's chest was clear, but it was apparent to me that his increasing confusion was due to his opiate use.

We had the same conversation I had already had with him many times over the last year. I told him that we needed to reduce his medication. We had tried to reduce his treatment before, but it had always been unsuccessful. Every time, this pain would rise up, a many-headed serpent, consuming him and putting him in bed, screaming, for days on end.

There are many protocols and theories in managing opiate reduction and withdrawal. Most agree that for patients such as Jasper, success relies on his engagement in the process. At that moment, this was something we did not have. His pain control and mental health were just not stable enough. A combined pain and addiction clinic would have been ideal, but this did not exist so we did not have that option. We had to wait it out, hoping that with time and continued support and therapy, one day he would agree to try.

And in the end, that day did come – but at a massive cost.

*

Jake and Jasper went away to Paris for the weekend, leaving their friend Wilbur to take care of their flat. Wilbur headed out to a local nightclub, then brought some people back home. The drug- and alcohol-fuelled party that ensued was of epic proportions. In the middle of the mayhem, Wilbur disappeared into a bathroom and did not reappear for many hours.

There were a number of bathrooms in the flat, and so no one noticed he was missing. It wasn't until 6 a.m., when most of the guests had left and only a few stragglers remained, that people started looking for him. He was nowhere to be found, but one of the bathroom doors remained locked and there was no response from within. Paramedics were called, and the police forced the door.

Wilbur was dead. He had suffocated on the thick-pile carpet of the tastefully decorated bathroom several hours before. The post-mortem showed a hugely high level of one of Jasper's opiate medications in his bloodstream. After a lengthy inquest, the verdict was 'misadventure'.

Jake and Jasper were distraught. They had been very close to Wilbur; he had been a loyal and diligent friend through health and illness. Jasper became very low and Jake asked me to come to see them at their flat.

I buzzed at the front entrance and they let me in. I got in the elevator and went up to the sixth floor. Jasper was waiting for me as I emerged. He was wearing a purple dressing gown and had a glass of wine in a crystal glass in one hand, despite it being 10.30 in the morning. He burst into tears when he saw me and bent his head against my shoulder, sobbing. I put my arm around him and patted his closely shorn head and thick, tattooed neck. We stayed like that for a few minutes, until someone needed to get into the lift.

The apartment door was open behind Jasper and we went in. Jake was standing in the entrance hall in a matching purple dressing gown. We had a group hug. While they both wept, I worked hard to compose my face as I took in the flat. At first glance, it was a beautiful, light, modern apartment, elegantly furnished. But as I studied the ornaments and pictures in more detail, it became harder and harder not to recoil in shock.

Massive marble penises were sat on a side table. I hastily averted my gaze, but found myself looking straight up the dilated anus of a young man in an enlarged, framed, close-up photograph on the wall. Moving away from that, I spotted a large oil painting in a thick gold mount. Initially it seemed like a fairly safe Rubens-style painting – until the detail revealed a much more carnal scene. I looked away again to a wooden carving on the dresser – a tribal man with an extended appendage protruding into the mouth of a kneeling figure.

'You're the first woman to have ever been in this flat,' Jake sobbed, as they showed me to a seat. I studiously looked out of the window for the rest of my visit.

We managed to have a productive conversation in spite of the distractions. As a result of Wilbur's death, both told me that they were now committed to reducing Jasper's opiate use. Perhaps this was due to a newfound fear of death, or maybe it was the change of perspective that being close to death can give a person. I wasn't sure, but whatever it was, it gave Jasper the conviction he needed. We agreed on a plan. But before that, they invited me to Wilbur's cremation the following week.

I knew it meant a lot to them, so I went. I arrived early. It was a beautiful day and there were lots of flowers blooming. I sat on a wooden bench outside the main crematorium building and waited. The priest arrived and we chatted idly about the weather and business. After about twenty minutes, a taxi pulled up and Jake and Jasper got out. They were in a sort of uniform of respect for the relationship they had had with Wilbur, and both wore maroon DM boots and stonewashed, skin-tight jeans, with white T-shirts underneath green bomber jackets, which had Union Jacks sewn onto their backs. Their heads were freshly shaved.

The priest led them to the coffin in the crematorium, which had been draped with a Union flag. Jasper, Jake and I sat on the front row of the wooden benches. We were the only people there. They insisted I sat in the middle.

We listened to the priest's short sermon, and then the shrill tones of Kate Bush's 'Running Up That Hill' filled the silence as the coffin moved into the furnace. The priest stood, head bowed with respect, while Jasper and Jake reminisced in graphic detail about the 'best times' they had had with Wilbur. Many of the activities they mentioned I would not have thought anatomically possible. They talked across me, remembering particular club nights and an extraordinarily active country walk. I have not been able to listen to 'Running Up That Hill' in the same way since.

Jasper's subsequent withdrawal from opiates tested both our resolves. He could tolerate only a very slow withdrawal from his medication which, in the end, took almost three years from start to finish. He fought the process of withdrawal at times, and he lied and hid medication, but Jake was constant and committed, refusing to collude with him until we gradually got him down to a single opiate, a fentanyl patch, which was the hardest part to withdraw from. Fentanyl is a synthetic variant of morphine, but many hundreds of times stronger, which makes it extremely addictive. Nowadays we only use it for patients with terminal illness.

On one occasion, Jake came home to find Jasper unconscious, having sucked the medication out of one of the patches and imbibed the equivalent of three days' worth of fentanyl in one hit. This nearly killed him, and he was hospitalised for several days. He then moved from patches to tablets, and finally to tiny amounts of opiate in liquid form.

The most extraordinary thing during this process was that Jasper's pain did not come back. The back pain he had suffered for years was gone. Nowadays, when he gets distressed or tired, he says he feels it at a low level – a dull reminder of another time. He works hard on his mental health. He sleeps and eats well. He barely drinks alcohol, and he meditates daily. He has changed his emotional state dramatically and this has changed his pain.

It is still hard to know what Jasper's pain might have been caused by. Was it the combination of deep emotional trauma and some bone degeneration in his spine? I'm pretty sure it was down to a variety of reasons that were difficult to pick apart. I think we can be confident, however, that his emotional state and his belief structure played a big part in it.

*

Ben the acupuncturist saw Troy for two months, and treated his chronic back and pelvic pain with acupuncture. Then he handed over his care to another of our therapists, Jess. The process was gradual, but as time went by, I found the outcome quite remarkable. Slowly, Troy was able to reduce his opiate medication and, finally, free himself of it. He was steadily strengthening his wellbeing. The process was fragile and precarious, requiring constant effort and attention. But Jess seemed to be keeping him stable. Then there was a major turning point – the discovery of the Brighton Table Tennis Club.

The Brighton Table Tennis Club opened in 2007. Shortly after we had started the practice, one of its founders, Tim Holten, had come along to see me. He had heard about our approach to health. His passion and enthusiasm were instantly infectious.

'Table tennis is so brilliant for anyone, anyone!' He sat in my consulting room, leaning forward and gesticulating with his arms.

'You can play in a wheelchair, you can play with one leg or one arm. It is excellent for strengthening hand-eye coordination after a stroke or in patients with Parkinson's or movement disorders. We have several incredible players with Down's syndrome and it's just *so much fun*! And, oh yes – we are also a sanctuary for refugees and asylum seekers!'

Tim was so persuasive that I found myself agreeing to install a large table tennis table in the waiting room. Gary swiftly pointed out the obvious health and safety issues of this and we had to drop the plan, but I visited their club in a converted bingo hall in Kemptown and I was immediately sold on it. The kindness of the place was almost palpable. As well as being serious in their sporting achievements, and competing on the national and international stage, they were also fundamentally inclusive, welcoming anyone who might be in need of a bit of extra support. The staff were like a loving and warm family with an overarching purpose, and Troy found his people here. He became a regular visitor, playing table tennis himself, helping out and enjoying the feeling of belonging.

When I started out on my journey at the practice, this was the kind of outcome I had hoped might be possible. And here it was. Troy's pain receded, and his progress was testimony to the success of the unconventional medical route he had taken. I was amazed and delighted. The work we were doing seemed truly worthwhile.

CHAPTER 7

Ethics

How does a doctor decide what is in a patient's interests? This can be a testing and challenging question. It's made harder when you realise that what the patient wants might be totally different to what you yourself would want in that situation.

Seeing the world through someone else's eyes, and wanting what they would want for themselves, can present serious challenges. It doesn't always feel like a kind and gentle process. It can even be shocking. Certainly, few patients in my own experience have been more challenging than Nancy.

Nancy was a slight woman; she had blondish hair, which fell in short curls around her face. She might have had a pretty face once, but years of trauma and abuse were stamped onto her, scarring her skin and deadening her eyes. Eyes can tell you a lot about a person. They are said to be the windows to the soul. In Nancy's case, the blinds were down. She operated on a thin veneer of emotion; most of her feelings appeared to be locked deep down beneath a hard, protective layer. Sometimes a chance comment or look would pierce this layer and release the boiling lava of pain and fury that churned beneath. She was certainly not the sort of person you would want to meet on a dark street at night.

Nancy had had four children over the course of her thirty-two years, all of whom had been removed from her care by social services.

She loved them all fiercely, but was gripped in a vicious cycle of recreational drug use, addiction and rehabilitation that prevented her from being able to care for them. In the absence of being able to be with her children, her current all-consuming love was for her dog, a rottweiler called Lola. She was a tough, loyal, strong character with a propensity for sudden violent outbursts – much like her owner.

Nancy first came to see me as she was determined to have some involvement in her youngest daughter's life after years of being separated from her. The baby had been taken from her by social services from birth. Knowing that social services would be waiting for her at the hospital, Nancy had planned to deliver her at a friend's flat, but the friend had lost their nerve at the last minute and called the paramedics. It was a good thing they did as Nancy's labour was obstructed and both she and her baby nearly died. She was rushed into hospital, where her daughter was born by caesarean section and taken away shortly afterwards.

Over the course of her life, Nancy had been forced to live on the outskirts of society. She did not have the tools to engage. She was used to being attacked, by people and by 'the system'. I once confided in her that sometimes I was scared walking home at night. Nancy had leant in towards me in a rare moment of connectedness and said, 'Doc, you gotta walk down that street like you own it.'

I had been seeing Nancy for over a year to take blood and urine samples and send them for drugs testing, as well as to offer her therapy. The judge had mandated this in an effort to address her problems after it was ruled that she was 'unstable'. Seeing a psychiatrist, or having any sort of long-term meaningful therapy, is not possible on the NHS. Six sessions of CBT is the only provision. That is pretty much it. Nancy had to make do with me, and if she came weekly, she'd be allowed supervised visits with her daughter.

I had been a GP for two years at this point. I'd read a book called *The GP's Guide to Ten-Minute Mental Health Consultations*. The basic message of this book was that you could not really do very much in ten minutes. So it was better not to try, for fear of unleashing any demons in the first five minutes of a consultation that you might not be able to pack away again in the second five minutes. I took this advice to heart: I certainly didn't feel like I would be capable of packing away the demons that I suspected lurked behind the firmly closed blinds of Nancy's eyes.

Fortunately, Nancy didn't really have any interest in talking to me. So, most of the time we just talked about her dog. Lola came everywhere with her; she was a scary-looking rottweiler but she gave her mistress the sort of unconditional love she had never experienced before. She defended Nancy, guarded her, doted on her. She sat outside the toilet when she was in there. She rested her head on Nancy's knee when she watched TV, and slept at the foot of her bed.

'How are the two of you doing?' I asked her at the start of one consultation. Nancy never said very much and today was going to be no exception. She looked at me with her still, dead eyes.

'Okay, doc.'

'Feeling okay?'

'Yeah.'

'What's happening right now? What's happened to you today?'

I knew I wasn't going to get much out of her. She told me slowly, but not unwillingly, about where she'd been that morning with Lola.

'Waiting for you outside, is she?'

I saw a glimmer of warmth cross her face.

'Yeah – she is.'

'Well, that's good. You'd better go and get her, then.'

Their relationship worked for her in a way that therapy never could have done. I supposed that somewhere deep in her childhood she had been significantly betrayed and let down. Here, finally, was a recipient of her love who was never going to do that to her, and who she could love and nurture in a way that she hadn't been able to do for her own children. I watched her leave my consulting room, then pictured her making her way to the railings and unfastening Lola's leash. I knew that she'd be overjoyed to see her.

Together, the two of them were happy.

*

Aretta, one of the local district nurses, was on the phone. She sounded very worried.

'It's Ted,' she explained quickly. 'He was spending the afternoon at the Dragon Inn – same as every other afternoon – but this time he fell off his stool and he couldn't get up.'

'Something more serious than just too much ale, I suppose?' I questioned her. I knew all about Ted's drinking. He sat on the stool at the corner of the bar at the Dragon Inn every day from 2 p.m. until it closed at 11.30 p.m., and then he tottered home. All the rich, close relationships of his life were there, in particular with the different bar staff, the pub owner, Golden Virginia tobacco, and ale.

'I'm afraid so. The Royal Surrey X-rayed him. Then they wanted a closer look, so they did an MRI. It's bad news.'

'How bad?'

'Terminal metastatic lung cancer. He's palliative, I'm afraid. There's a DNACPR in place.'

A DNACPR is a set of instructions. It stands for Do Not Attempt Cardio-Pulmonary Resuscitation. It essentially means that if the patient's heart were to stop, resuscitation would not be attempted. Doctors make the decision, usually in discussion with family members. It's based on the probability that, first of all, resuscitation isn't likely to work, and, and, secondly, that even if it did, it wouldn't work for long and the trauma and violence of the procedure would harm the patient for barely any gain.

Ted was infused with antibiotics and fluids, and then sent home. Macmillan nurses and district nurses went around to see him. Now, as Aretta explained, they were concerned that he was unsafe there. They wanted a doctor to review him. He needed, they said, to be moved to a nursing home for the short amount of his life that remained to him.

I walked down the Lanes to his house. He lived in the basement flat of a tall terraced house on one of the smaller squares in Brighton near the sea. It was a bright, clear day and there was a cold crispness in the air that reminded me of being in snow-tipped French mountains.

I walked down narrow, treacherous stone stairs to the basement door. It was in a state of disrepair. I knocked and waited for a long time. It seemed like forever, but eventually there was a movement and the sound of the lock being turned. A tiny figure opened the door and let me in. Ted was wearing faded pyjamas with some sort of stripe on them and a lot of tying around the waist. I stepped into his house, and for a moment I felt like I had walked into his lung.

The bronchial corridor was narrow and dimly lit and the walls were stained dark brown with nicotine and tarry deposits. The air was close and heavy with stagnant molecules. I took in shallow breaths through my nose to filter out as much debris as possible. Ted disappeared off down the pulmonary labyrinth like a wizened hobbit inhabiting his own insides. I followed him.

We turned the corner where the corridor widened, alveoli-like, into a room. At the end of the room there was a small window, which should have opened onto the freshly oxygenated world outside. But dark net curtains hung against the yellowing panes, blocking the exchange of light and air.

Ted got onto his bed and lay there, the walk having exhausted him.

I sat on the bed, perching with one buttock rested, the other supported by my tensed right thigh. This would be a test of my squat strength.

I waited for him to speak. It took a while.

'I don't want to go into a hospital,' he said. 'I know that's why you're here, but I don't want to go. This place doesn't look like much to you, but it's my home. I want to die here.'

I looked at him, lying in his tobacco-saturated world. Then, somehow, I came to be holding his hand and making a low 'umming' noise in my throat. His room, his house, its walls and ceilings, his bed, his clothes – they all seemed to be made of the same yellowed organic matter as he was. Of course he didn't want to be whipped out to a nursing home, popped into a starched, clean bed under a bright white strip light, surrounded by kindly tutting, chlorinated staff.

'I understand,' I replied. 'Really, I do.'

Most of the front-line staff who attend to patients in their homes understand. But what scares all of us was perfectly articulated by Aretta when I called her again after my visit.

'But he can't stay there,' she said sharply, panic rising in her voice. 'What if he falls? What if he cracks his head and dies like that? What will they say?'

I knew what she meant. *They* would say, 'Who left him in an unsafe flat? Who let him fall and die on the floor in a pool of his own blood in a stinking hovel? It's disgusting!' *They* would say 'uncaring and *negligent*'.

A death like that would have to go to the coroner and questions would be asked. Blame would be cast. Someone would have to pay. It would be so much easier for all of us to have Ted tucked safely in a sanitised bed with the fall-guard up. Then no one could question that we did the right thing.

However, in my experience there are things that matter more to people than safety. There are many things that people are willing to take risks for, to die for: love, justice, peace, familiarity. Meaning and purpose are our biggest driving forces, not health and safety. Yet it is health and safety that govern all our institutionalised, decision-making tools. We are taught to ask people what they want, what they value... but *acting* on that, going against protocol and National Institute for Health and Care Excellence (NICE) guidance, is a completely different matter.

There is a deep underlying assumption that a doctor must ask patients what they want, and if their answers do not fit with what is considered 'best practice', then the clinician must persuade and educate them. We are taught that, in the end, the patient will see sense and come around. If, after all that, they still don't want to obey protocol, then the frequent conclusion is that they might be lacking in mental capacity or, even worse, just plain difficult – and then there's nothing more we can do for them.

'I think he should stay at home,' I said down the phone to my nursing colleague. 'I'll go and see him tomorrow and talk to him again. Let's leave him for the moment. Don't worry – I'm the one who'll be going to the Coroner's Court, not you.'

She would have to talk to her team, she told me. She would document all this. She clearly wasn't happy.

There is a fear that runs through the decision-making of healthcare workers. It's a fear of being seen to do the wrong thing, and it's become so powerful that it often prevents us from doing the right thing. It is a dark shadow that hints at litigation, investigation, inquiry and humiliation. It is a fear that does not serve us or our patients well.

In the end, Ted died that night in his familiar, filthy, tarry bed. We'd taken a risk to make it happen, but I think we'd made the right call.

*

Identifying a patient's best interests is at its most challenging when the person has lost some or all cognitive function, especially when their relatives disagree with each other. Having dementia does not necessarily mean you don't have capacity. You may still be able to give a clear and reliable opinion. You may not, however, fully understand the implications of it. You may even welcome your hallucinations.

My patient, Annie, had a remarkable ability to sound plausible even in the most unlikely circumstances. This made her diagnosis of dementia tricky.

For a long time, I believed her seven sisters were all still alive and living in Aylesbury. They were a wonderful sisterhood. As the youngest, she had watched their teenage antics from various vantage points, hiding on the stairs above the landing, or in the potting shed behind the 'kissing swing'.

Theirs sounded like an idyllic life in a big rambling house in the Somerset countryside with a slightly crazed father who spent most of his time in his study. While she talked, I populated the scene with devilishly handsome *Pride and Prejudice*-type characters in britches and tailcoats wooing the sisters, whom I imagined in bonnets and flowing dresses. Agnes, the eldest, was overbearing and bossed the other sisters around, a characteristic which Sally and Constance had always resented.

Annie spoke to them every day – except that they were all dead. I was quite shocked when I found out. Her extreme dementia had been covered by her well-meaning youngest daughter, Janine, who still lived with her; Annie in her eighties, Janine in her early fifties. Janine was obsessed with Annie's diet and with her duty to care for her mother as her mother had cared for her. She was definitely on the autistic spectrum, though no doctor had made this diagnosis.

Theirs was an impassioned and, I feared, sometimes violent relationship. Janine had been terribly bullied as an 'odd' child in the 1970s. Annie's older children were super-intelligent and attractive, from a different father who had left just before Janine was born. They had pretty much left home while she was growing up, and Annie felt they had never had any real connection with their youngest sibling. She was of unknown origin, Annie told me, with a twinkle in her eye.

Sometimes Annie would come into the surgery with bruises on her arms where she told me she had fallen, but the bruising was not consistent with her story. This could have been down to her failing memory, but neighbours complained about arguments and loud noises they heard coming from the house. Sometimes Janine would attend consultations with her and railroad any discussion with her extensive diarising of Annie's diet and pain and lapses of memory. She refused to accept Annie's dementia diagnosis, even when her symptoms were very bad and her cognitive function severely impaired. She would not allow the word to be used around her for fear it would upset her.

Janine was incredibly attentive to her mother, administering increasingly strict food portions of reducing quantities. Her research, she said, had led her to believe that more and more foods were 'poison' and damaging to her mother's health. In spite of not knowing where she was or what time of day it was or even what year, Annie had total and utter clarity about her children and what she felt about them. And she adored Janine.

Janine needed her, and more than anything in the world, Annie wanted to be with Janine too. Annie alluded to multiple instances where she had defended Janine from the sneers and derision of her peers and their families. She would have laid down her life for her, she would have taken the harshest of punishments for her, even from Janine herself. I grew increasingly concerned that Janine was doing just that.

Annie's weight was decreasing and her hip pain was worsening. Janine was refusing to give her painkillers as she felt they were toxic and could make her worse. She had a point: sometimes these drugs can increase confusion and cause other side effects. Most interventions and medical solutions require a fine balance that a patient must discuss carefully with their doctor to counterbalance risk and gain, harm and cure, relieving suffering and shortening life, non-maleficence and beneficence.

The kinds of decisions that need to be made in order to achieve this balance must be individual and well informed. They cannot be the stuff of guidelines or protocols.

I knew what might happen if I involved social services with Annie's case. I would bring Annie to their attention as a vulnerable adult, and kind, well-meaning social workers would come and deliberate her case, trying to help. They would seek to push Janine to behave in a more socially acceptable and normal way. As a result, she would become more anxious and controlling as what she feared the most (not being able to take care of her mother) started to become a reality. Annie would end up in a nursing home away from Janine, possibly even with a restriction order limiting their contact. Although this would keep her physically safe, I was unsure that this was what Annie would have chosen for herself.

Every time I asked her what she wanted in terms of her care, she was quite clear she wanted to stay with Janine. She brought meaning to her life. Then she would tell me about the conversation she had just had with her sister Constance or about how bossy Agnes was being.

I agonised over this. I spoke to colleagues and there was no consensus. I desperately wanted to take Annie's case to an ethics committee, but the only one I knew reviewed clinical trials and took about two years to do it. In situations like this, GPs need guidance not just from experienced ethicists, but from philosophers, anthropologists, writers and humanitarians to help us navigate the moral maze.

In caring for Annie, my dilemma was this: did I set in motion a train of events that would potentially take the meaning from her life to protect her safety and health, or did I let her stay living with her daughter, potentially allowing her to suffer at her misguided but loving hands?

In the end, her neighbours made the decision for me. There was a particularly disturbed night during which voices were loudly raised. A report went out to social services and the inevitable train of events occurred.

We find it difficult as human beings not to think in binary terms and tend to weigh up decisions on a dichotomous scale of good and evil. In the eyes of the social services, Janine was therefore cast as evil, and there was no scope in our care or judicial system to accommodate and adequately recognise the complexity of Annie's situation, or her daughter's motivation.

At the time of writing, Annie has been living in a nursing home for two years. I have just got back from visiting her. She has gained weight and has no bruises, but she barely speaks or gets out of bed. She has completely withdrawn from the world since leaving Janine. When I arrived late last night, a small, efficient nurse let me in from the windy, rainy night and showed me to Annie's room. Annie was lying on a bed in the half-dark.

Care staff had noticed that Annie's foot was hot and swollen.

'I am sorry to wake you, Annie. The doctor's here,' said the small, efficient nurse.

Annie's clear, confident voice rose up from a pile of old-fashioned covers on the bed. I was unable to see any of her at all at this point, as her head was under the eiderdown.

'Don't be silly,' she said. 'I love doctors.'

'Hi, Annie. It's me, Laura, Dr Marshall-Andrews – do you remember me?'

'Of course I remember you,' said the pile of covers. 'You've grown your hair.' It was a lucky guess for someone lying under several thick blankets with their eyes closed.

'Yes,' I said.

I kept talking to her as I examined her, and she kept her eyes firmly closed.

'Is everything okay?' she asked.

'Yes, Annie, you just have an infection in your foot.'

'Oh, I thought so. I keep in very good health, you see. I still play tennis every day.'

I look down at her wasted muscles and the fixed deformities of her limbs, as she lay in the corner of this dingy room, playing out the scenes from her past life like a movie in her mind.

If you're lucky enough to have had a happy life, then sometimes dementia can even be beautiful, as it rewinds images from your past. It is your favourite film. In the end, it is our memories we are left with, so it's up to us to make sure they are as good as possible.

*

I first met Mary in the waiting room of the practice. She was in her mid-forties, and she was larger than life. She had the stigmata of drink etched on her face, not to the extent of actual alcoholism or illness, but enough to know it played more than a bit-part in her day-to-day routine.

She looked fun: the kind of person you would like to sit next to at a dinner party. She was talking away to a fellow patient on the colourful plastic chairs, with the light from the large window behind her. There was a beauty to her wildly animated face flashing behind her gesticulating arms. I called her name and she stood up without stopping her flow of words, walking towards me while effortlessly moving into a different conversation.

At the time, I wondered if she ever stopped talking. Over the ensuing years, we were destined to have many meetings, and throughout them all there would only be a few moments that brought her to a halt. The last of these was her death.

I was prepared for consultations with patients like this. 'The garrulous patient' is an Objective Structured Clinical Examination station during medical training. OSCEs are actor-led consultations during which student doctors are examined. 'The garrulous patient' situation tested our skills at containing and communicating effectively with someone who talks incessantly. It was by far the hardest test and almost everyone failed it.

Faced with Mary, I attempted several of the very basic skills I had acquired during this training, but they were no match for her. About an hour later, she left my consulting room and moved straight into conversation with our deputy practice manager, who happened to be standing outside my door.

I was left slightly unsure of why she had attended the surgery that day. But I did now know an awful lot about her life and family. And it was fascinating and enthralling and tragic.

Mary had spent most of her adult life desperately trying to extricate her younger sister, Shannon, from an abusive relationship that had kept her under coercive control for the best part of a decade. Over the years Shannon had withdrawn further and further into herself; Mary and her husband had done everything they could to help her leave but, in the end, Shannon's inability to admit to herself the severity of the situation that she was in thwarted their attempts. It was only when Mary's husband passed away after a sudden, tragic heart attack, and Shannon began to realise that Mary needed her sister just as much as she needed her, that Shannon began to listen to Mary. Mary found a flat that would be big enough to house her, her two small children and Shannon, and organised to steal Shannon away in the middle of the night on a rare occasion when her partner was away. Together, the family made it to London.

For a few years, it looked as though their brave flight had paid off. They shared a flat in East London and then moved down to Brighton. The kids started at nursery and then primary school. Shannon worked from home cutting hair in their converted front room, and Mary got a job in a local upmarket clothes shop.

One day in the shower, Shannon noticed a small lump in her breast. She thought nothing of it, until it became a hardened red mass. She went to the GP and had a scan, which lit up 'like a Christmas tree'. There were multiple cancer deposits in her bones and lungs.

Shannon had cycles of chemotherapy and surgery and radiotherapy, and when these didn't work, she prepared to die, leaving Mary alone with her children once more.

It was ten years after this that I met Mary, that day in the waiting room. She had another partner by now, a delightful man who almost never spoke but was happy to listen to her. Her children were at secondary school. The eldest was about to sit his GCSEs. But Mary had just been diagnosed with breast cancer that had already spread to her bones and lungs. By the time I met her, she had been referred to the Marsden Hospital in London. She had had a double mastectomy, then several rounds of chemotherapy and radiotherapy.

We met every few months to review her cancer markers and discuss her consultations at the Marsden with her very eminent consultant and experienced team. For a while, the markers stayed down. Her scans showed stable disease in the bone and the lung 'nodule' had almost disappeared.

Then, horribly, slowly and cruelly, the cancer markers started to rise. The dark blot on her lung gained intensity and more patches appeared in her spine. It had seemed unthinkable that she would suffer the same fate as her sister, yet this was just what seemed to be happening.

She started attending my surgery on a weekly basis, emptying out her distress and fear into the tiny, airless consulting room. She was going to fight this thing, she said, and she was going to win.

One wintery day, she came in telling me that she was no longer going to attend her appointments at the Marsden.

'I can't cope with them telling me I am going to die all the time,' she said. 'I think it's worse than the cancer, worse than anything. Their words are killing me. I have to keep fighting this, I have to, I can't stop. You understand that, don't you?'

I listened to her. I agreed that no one knew what her story would be. No one knew exactly what would happen to her. Then I spoke to the team at the Marsden: kind, experienced nurses and seasoned oncologists. Their position was clear. She had to face her death. It was the only way for her.

They agreed there were examples of people who had survived her stage of disease, but they were very, very rare. There was no common thread among those cases. The causes of late or sudden remission of cancer are probably genetic, or due to a sudden switching-on of the host's immune system. These were not relevant to Mary's case. The Marsden team felt it was immoral to 'give her false hope'.

But Mary would not have it. She was not going to die from this disease, and she was not going to talk to anyone who told her she was. She felt betrayed by them, and abandoned.

I was conflicted by this situation. On the one hand, the Marsden's professionals were right: the chance was high that Mary would die, and so preparing and 'coming to terms with it' would help her and her family be at peace. It would also help us, as doctors and nurses, if she followed the standard pattern that other patients did. All our systems and funding streams are set up in NICE-guided channels and flow charts. These have been created to maximise cost-effective benefits, according to mass data from clinical trials.

But there were two things that bothered me. One: we could not be 100 per cent sure that she would not be one of the rare, extraordinary survival stories, and two: this was her journey to take, her life to live and death to die. Should we not be able to support her to do that in the manner of her choice, to die in the manner in which she had lived: bravely, heroically and embattled? She was not asking for expensive medication. She was asking for a different way of being spoken to. She was asking to be allowed to hold onto a tiny, thin, golden ember of hope.

I chose to stay with her on the path of her choice.

And so she embarked on a voyage through a plethora of high-promising alternative treatments. I endeavoured to keep an open mind towards the different pathways she explored, no matter how bizarre they seemed.

One day she came to see me to discuss a recent blood test and review her steadily reducing weight. She arrived in her usual manner, midway through a long conversation, which I felt sure she must have been having seamlessly for most of the day with varying participants. I gathered she was talking about a recent teaching from the Dalai Lama. Halfway through the conversation, while I was attempting to listen to her chest and take her blood pressure, she seemed to run out of steam. I looked up and took my stethoscope out of my ear. She sat there motionless, uncharacteristically silent. Then, 'Oh, fuck the Dalai Lama,' she said, and left.

She had the most incredible energy and put this down to drinking Irn-Bru – the drink 'made in Scotland from girders'. And even as her body wasted away, consumed by the ravenous cancer that was devouring her, she still had a vibrancy and shine that was more than Irn-Bru could have induced.

In the end, she became too weak to get to the surgery reliably, so I visited her in her flat. She was in bed and I sat at her side to examine her. Her muscle bulk had reduced so much that her ribs jutted clearly through her thin nightie. She was still talking. She was travelling up to London tomorrow, she said, to see a new private consultant who was trialling a new chemotherapy. She must have seen the horror in my face. Going to London? She could barely walk to the toilet.

'Don't you look at me like that,' she snapped. She didn't make it to London, but she died trying. She's not alone in that. People often die as they live, and that's their choice. We might want them tucked up in bed, accepting of death, but this may not be their character. So be it.

For my part, I mourned Mary. I had given so much of myself to her and to her family. I expected her partner and children to continue to see me and want to involve me in their lives. They didn't. I was just the doctor. Although sometimes it's painful, that is how it should be.

*

One dark, windy morning in February, I was walking to work along the seafront. The sea was unusually churning and restless. Enormous waves crashed onto the shingle, hurling pebbles onto the walkway. The wind picked up my scarf and pulled it tight around my neck. I turned into the Lanes, away from the wild weather and into the relative protection of the narrow streets.

As I approached the practice, I could see someone standing outside the front door. The door was open and other patients were filing in to collect prescriptions and bag early appointments. The figure was standing alert, to attention, waiting for something. As I got closer, I recognised Nancy and her partner, Dave. This was not Nancy's normal day to see me. As I got closer, she left Dave's side and ran towards me. I had not seen her like this before. There was a depth to her expression that was new. I took a moment to work it out: it was fear.

'I have to speak to you, doc, I know it's not my day but...' Her voice stopped short. Her eyes darted around, looking up the road and back down towards the sea.

'It's okay,' I replied trying to keep calm and not become infected by her contagious anxiety.

As we got closer to the entrance of the practice where Dave was still standing, I noticed he had damp sweat marks covering his top, and his trousers were soaked through.

'Come with me,' I said, and we walked into the practice, past the waiting room full of patients and straight up the stairs. I wasn't sure what had happened, but I didn't feel like booking an appointment for them both later in the day was the right option. There was a palpable urgency about them.

We entered my consultation room and Dave shut the door behind me and Nancy. He stood with his back pressed against the closed door, while I moved to turn on the computer and load up the system. He was breathing hard. Now that we were in a confined space, I could smell him. He smelt of sweat, alcohol and the sea. His lack of willingness to move from the door meant that, for the first time, I felt a pang of fear. Nancy was hovering close to him, unsure where to look, before she moved forward to speak to me. I gestured for the two of them to sit; Dave painstakingly peeled himself from the door and sat with Nancy in one of the seats next to me.

'We killed her,' she said, staring at me wildly. Then she burst into tears. Huge sobs wracked her body. 'We had to!' she cried. 'We had to!'

My mind whirred. I had no idea at all who she could mean. For a horrible moment I thought she might have meant her youngest child. I started rubbing her back, trying to calm her down. 'She bit a child. She bit a child on the leg,' Dave moaned.

Then it hit me like a stone. They had killed Nancy's dog. They had killed Lola.

'We didn't know what to do.' Dave was talking in a clear voice now. 'We had to tell you. You understand what Lola meant to Nancy. I didn't know how to do it.'

Slowly they explained what had happened. They had been having a pint together on the seafront the day before, after having walked Lola. She was lying at Nancy's feet, on guard, protecting her. A small child had stumbled over to speak to her mother. While her mother was talking to another table, the child had reached out to Lola, and as she did so, she had stumbled and fallen into the chair that Nancy was sitting on. Lola had registered an attack. She had risen up, snarling, and bitten the child's leg as she was trying to get back up.

In the chaos and screaming that ensued, Nancy and Dave grabbed Lola and dragged her away. They ran all the way back to their flat, half carrying her, half pulling her. They knew she would have to be put down. Together, they had reflected on the different ways they might be able to kill her as quickly and humanely as possible. They thought about poisoning her. They thought about suffocating her. At no point did it occur to them to take her to the vet. Such a rational and legitimate response was simply not in either of their make-up.

In the end, Nancy went to the butcher and bought a steak. She sat on the floor next to her and hugged and talked to her while she ate her last meal. They waited until the middle of the night, giving her as much love as they could, before they took her down to the beach, where they'd spent so many happy hours together. Dave waded out into the water with her as she was playing and drowned her, crying uncontrollably.

Someone must have seen them down by the sea. As they stumbled back across the beach, having had to commit their awful deed, they saw riot police making their way down to the place where Dave had got into the water with Lola. Nancy insisted that they turn and flee to the practice.

'They'll be here soon,' Dave said. 'Nance just wanted you to know.' He wiped his face with his hands and stood up. 'We're gonna go.'

He went over to the door and opened it. Crouched outside were three of my receptionists with their ears to the door. He looked back at me and smiled wryly. 'I guess everyone will know the truth now.' I nodded, unable to speak.

The police were outside when they left. Apparently they both got in the car peacefully. Dave was sentenced to several months' imprisonment for 'grievous harm to animals'. I don't think my statement to the police helped him and I don't think they thought it would. Nancy's lack of involvement in the murder didn't prevent her from having her contact from her daughter irrevocably removed by the court.

They wanted it known that they weren't the monsters people would think they were. They didn't live in a world of vets and process and procedure. They both lived in a violent, brutal world, so that was how they solved their problems – with violence. It wasn't right, but they had tried to do what seemed right. They wanted someone to know this: that Nancy had loved Lola, that it had been incredibly hard for them to kill her, but they had done what they thought was right in the kindest way they knew how.

CHAPTER 8

Power

I have become more and more aware as the years have gone by of the authority that medical professionals have. It's a humbling realisation. I believe that this authority should be used with the most careful thought, and maximum awareness of the patient and their feelings and needs.

Of course, it isn't always the case that we are figures of power and importance. In some respects, a doctor can become almost completely invisible. I once had a patient come to see me about a swollen knee. He was adamant he had seen me the previous week, but I really didn't remember him. When I looked back in the notes, it was in fact one of my colleagues he had seen. This would have been an understandable mistake had my colleague not been an elderly man on the brink of retirement, with a receding hairline and of rather portly stature. But his presence hadn't registered with the patient at all. Both of us were simply 'the doctor'.

But on other occasions, I have certainly experienced just how powerful a doctor's presence can be.

Peter was a local GP who retired just as I qualified. He had a loyal cohort of patients, whom he had seen through many of the milestones of their lives. He had provided comfort and reassurance through childhood illnesses, had been an impartial confidante for consultations around early sexual encounters, a shoulder to cry on when jobs or studies were tough. He had seen patients through pregnancies and childbirth, parental anxieties, divorces and deaths. He had dispensed medications and kindnesses. He had borne witness to their suffering and to their triumphs and helped them make sense of tragedies.

Throughout his long career, Peter had operated with absolute autonomy and did entirely what he and his patient considered best. He had never used a protocol or taken any exams in general practice. He'd faced no revalidation or appraisals. He did very little paperwork, and usually made it home for lunch and a quick prune of the roses. His surgeries would have had about ten to twelve patients, and he would have done several home visits in the morning. Those were the days, I am sometimes tempted to say.

If someone had a heart attack back then, they usually went to bed with an aspirin as there was very little else that could be done. But the vast majority of patients he saw survived, and they all loved him. There was, and still is, a calmness about him. To be around him, one must slow down and match his kind, deliberate pace.

One of his patients moved to my surgery when he left practice and retired. Her name was Penny. She was in her seventies and lived in a glamorous flat overlooking the sea. It had high ceilings and tall, graceful windows that opened onto a small wrought-iron balcony. Penny had had many husbands, who beamed out from black-and-white photos in silver frames on the dresser and mantelpiece. But it was clear to me that her real and unrequited love was her GP.

'Where is Peter now?' she would implore me. 'Oh, he was such a marvellous man.' Her eyes would fill with tears.

She had been seeing another GP who had changed her medication. This had had a disastrous effect on Penny. Now she was a 'ball of nerves'. She had terrible pains in her chest and abdomen. When I visited her, she was reclining on a type of chaise lounge and declared she was unable to move. Her symptoms were vague and confusing, not typical of any one pathological process.

'I must see Peter!' she cried. 'I can't go on like this – it's intolerable!'

I knelt down next to her and took her hands. She had lost much of the bulk in the tiny muscles between the prominent metacarpal bones. Blue veins spread out across the backs of them, like tendrils of a jungle vine. Her nails were perfectly manicured, with thickly painted pink enamel. Jewels flashed from every finger. Emeralds from Ronnie, a sapphire from darling Paul, and a white-gold ring encrusted with tiny diamonds from her last husband, whom she referred to as Duke.

'The pain is unbearable,' she whispered. 'I can hardly breathe. I don't think I have long now.'

I listened to her heart and chest. Her pulse was strong and regular. Her chest was clear and her heart sounds were normal. Her blood pressure was excellent, and her skin was well perfused and pink. She looked in remarkably good health. I sat back down and watched her for a minute. She looked at me, terrified.

'Is it very bad?' she asked. 'I don't know why they stopped my special pill. It is very important to me. Peter said it would keep me well and calm me down. I simply must have it back. Please, doctor, please.'

I assumed that her 'special pill' must have been some sort of high-strength barbiturate tranquiliser. These used to be handed out fairly liberally to elderly ladies of an anxious disposition. I looked back through her notes, but the only medication she had been on was a very low-dose diuretic called bendroflumethiazide, rarely prescribed nowadays. It is generally recognised as having no medical value whatsoever. I called Peter on my mobile from the corridor and asked him about it.

'Oh, yes,' he said with a chuckle. 'That worked wonders! It's all about the way you give it! Prescribe her an anti-anxiety medication if you want,' he laughed, 'but it will cause her much more harm.'

I had to admit that he was right. Most of the anti-anxiety medication we have nowadays causes significant side effects. However, I had been schooled in evidence-based medicine, in an era when randomised controlled trials were king. It went against my training to prescribe a drug I knew to be worthless.

'Is it worthless, though?' Peter asked me, and he told me a story from his early career that had changed the way he thought about medicine.

Back then, he had been the GP to a local nursing home. They had about a hundred residents, making it a moderate-sized home. Most nursing homes of this size would call him out almost weekly for various minor illnesses and requests. However, this particular nursing home had only called him out once in the past year. He started to wonder about this, and looked up some of their statistics. Their death rate was unusually low. The frequency of hospital admissions was also significantly lower than usual. There was something interesting going on here, something that meant residents were surviving well with much less medical intervention. It seemed worth investigating, so he went to talk to the matron.

Matron was a brusque, no-nonsense woman, always dressed in uniform, with an air of ruthless discipline about her. She did not suffer fools gladly. When Peter explained that he was interested in how she managed her clients so effectively and hardly ever had need to call him in or send anyone to hospital, she looked at him over the top of her spectacles and snorted.

'It's very simple,' she said. 'We have the "step ladder". If anyone has pain or feels a bit unwell, we give them a multivitamin in a soft, clear capsule. Most of the time, they feel a lot better. If that doesn't work, then they progress to the fizzy vitamin C tablet. Most things are cured by that and it can be repeated as necessary. If after all that they are still in pain or feeling unwell, then they get the blue-and-white capsule. That's paracetamol.'

Then she paused, before continuing solemnly: 'It is *extremely* rare that we need to use the large red tablet.'

'What is the large red tablet?' Peter asked her, transfixed.

Matron leaned in and whispered: 'Ibuprofen, 200mg. Never fails.' And then she laughed and said, 'It's all about the way you give it!'

When Peter told me this story, I was torn between reporting Matron for unethical behaviour, and nominating her for some sort of Nobel Prize.

All this flashed through my mind as I sat there wondering what I should do for my patient Penny, suffering terrible pain and discomfort and pleading for a course of treatment that – from a scientific point of view – I knew to be of no value whatsoever. Finally, I made my decision.

I went back into the room where Penny was waiting for me. I sat down and took her hand in mine. I told her I had spoken to Peter and would be reinstating her medication immediately. She thanked me.

Penny lived a full and active life well into her eighties, sustained and invigorated every day by a low, regular dose of what was considered by conventional medical wisdom to be a totally ineffective medicine. Of course, looked at another way, it might be perceived as wholly effective. From Penny's point of view, this was a vital and wonderful treatment. And shouldn't it be Penny's experience that matters the most?

*

I was on call again. Being the on-call doctor means you take the immediate and urgent calls and deal with them as they come in. It usually means a busy day and requires careful priority setting. That day the telephone list was already nearly full, and it was only 9.30 a.m.

I flicked down through the names and the receptionist's notes next to them: Allen, fifty-six years old, flu symptoms, one week, thinks he needs antibiotics; Lucinda, forty, mental health issues; Matthew, twenty-five, anxious and suicidal; Frank, ninety-six, difficulty breathing.

I chose Frank and called the nursing home number. A nurse answered the phone. She had a slight accent – Spanish, I think. She knew Frank. I heaved a sigh of relief – no need to hold the line for precious minutes while someone else is found, watching more patients' names being added to my steadily growing call list.

She told me that Frank had been visited two days ago by the out-of-hours doctor. A chest infection was diagnosed and antibiotics prescribed. Now she felt that he was worse. She thought he might be dying.

I looked down his past medical history. Not much really, for ninety-six years old. A bit of high blood pressure, mild COPD (chronic obstructive pulmonary disease – the smoker's disease). Just on inhalers and a few blood-pressure medications. I noted the title of 'Reverend' in front of his name.

I agreed to go up there to see him. If he died, I would need to have done so to be able to produce a death certificate. I had never met him before; he'd registered a few months ago, probably when he was moved to the nursing home. I asked the nurse about relatives. No one – just a friend who lived 300 miles away, Terry. He was on his way down.

Frank and Terry – names from another era, when priests and doctors still smoked and said what the hell they liked. No CCG, no CQC, no Medicines Management Team. I wonder if it's better now, or worse.

I sent a message on the internal practice notification system. It went out to everyone – thirty-four people. 'Sorry – got to go on a visit. Back ASAP.'

When I reached the nursing home, Frank was lying in bed. His body was skeletal. His skin hung in dry, thin folds off the narrow bones in his arms and legs. His ribs were well demarcated and almost stationary. His eyes were closed, and his head turned to one side. For a moment, I thought he was dead. Then I noticed the soft, almost infinitesimal movement of his chest. The nurse stood next to me, looking expectantly. I knelt by the bed and gently touched Frank's forehead. He opened his eyes and looked straight at me.

Watery, blue, weak eyes. Eyes tired of seeing, worn out with the light. Deep in them, there was a tiny spark. I started talking to him. The nurse tried to put a hearing aid in his ears, but it made the most appalling noise and we all recoiled.

I picked up a pen and wrote on a large piece of paper: *Hello Reverend, I am the doctor.* His eyes moved over it, and he blinked, slowly taking in the words. So slowly that at one point I again wondered if he had died. But then he turned his head to me and nodded. Then a wonderful smile crept over his face. I smiled back and took his hand. We sat together, both taking in the situation. I reached into my bag for my stethoscope, pulse oximeter, sphygmomanometer and thermometer. I went through the motions I have been through many thousands of times. I listened to his chest, took his blood pressure and his temperature, and read his oxygen saturations.

His blood pressure was unmeasurable, pulse thready, temperature low and oxygen sats 80 per cent, but the trace was poor and unreliable.

I picked up the pen and wrote, *Are you comfortable?* He paused to read and then nodded. I asked the question again in a different way to check his comprehension. *Do you have any pain?* He shook his head.

I turned to the nurse, about to issue my diagnosis and plan, when Frank suddenly made an odd, guttural noise. I leaned closer to him and realised he was trying to speak. The wasted muscles between his ribs were barely able to create enough power to force out the breath. He tried again. I bent forward and put my ear close to his lips.

I just about made out the words 'Am I...?' and again, 'Am I...?' I pulled back. He was surely going to ask me whether he was dying. I composed my face to an expression of sympathy and understanding, preparing to reply in the affirmative.

'Am I... okay?' he whispered.

I was somewhat taken aback by this question. I supposed the short answer was 'No'. By most normal parameters, Frank was about as far from okay as it is possible to be. My knees were starting to feel uncomfortable on the hard floor. I reached out and held onto his hand, which lay over his chest. He looked like an angular, crooked bird, injured and helpless, watching me, waiting for my verdict.

'Yes,' I replied, suddenly feeling a huge amount of love and affection for his intense vulnerability. 'Yes.' I nodded, and slowly stroked his forehead for a few minutes. He smiled slightly, a minuscule upturning at the sides of his mouth.

I barely made it to the end of the road before the nurse called me back to say that he had died.

I often wonder what he meant by that question. And what I meant by my answer. Could he really have been so delusional that he thought there was any chance he was 'okay'? And was I colluding in that delusion?

Or was he in fact okay? I think now that in many ways, as he lay there, peaceful and calm after a long and varied life, he was completely okay. More okay than I have known yet, or could imagine. Perhaps at that moment of ending and utter hopelessness, there is absolute acceptance and peace. There is no more struggle or aspiration or worry or dread.

It's over. You can relax now. It's okay.

So it was with Frank. He was seeking permission to die. And I, as his doctor, had the power to give it – the power to let him go in peace. He'd lived long, and I hope that he had been fulfilled. Certainly, whatever had happened to him had brought him to an ending without fear.

PART 3

Fighting for survival

CHAPTER 9

Error

'We are all wrong no matter how good we are. We need people around us to tell us. Be open to suggestions. Listen to your team. Step up and lead.'
— MARTIN BROMILEY

Diane had spent her life working for the British Council. She had worked in Ethiopia, Ghana and Gabon. Her small flat was a tasteful, if somewhat overcrowded, museum of beautiful and strange artefacts from her worldly travels.

She was highly organised and did not suffer fools gladly. She had dinner parties with learned people, and they discussed matters of ethics and colonialism. She was medium height and thin, with dark chestnut hair, even at sixty years old, which frizzed up and had to be smoothed over repeatedly with her hands.

Her eyes were bright and intense. There was something almost bird-like about her. She did not smile very often, so when she did you were hugely grateful for it. It felt like a window briefly being flung open to reveal a warm, light-filled interior, only to be quickly shut again in case you saw too much of the scene inside.

She was irritated by an incessant drip of thin mucus from the back of her nasal passages down her throat. This is a condition called postnasal drip, and causes a tiresome cough. She had been to see everyone we could both think of, and she had done everything doctors recommended. Eventually, she went to an eminent respiratory consultant at the Brompton Chest Hospital. After much imaging and some trial and error, they discovered that a daily dose of a specific antihistamine and adrenaline-based medication might help.

Diane was very happy on this medication for several years. She could entertain and give talks without a persistent eye-watering cough interrupting her flow. Occasionally she would come to see me with some minor health complaint. At the end of the consultation I was usually in possession of new insight into Ghana's tribal community, say, or Ethiopia's rock-hewn churches.

But one day, she arrived bursting with anger. When Charlotte, the receptionist, recorded her arrival, she noticed this and helpfully tapped a quick message to warn me. It popped up on my screen, and as I waited for Diane to make her way to my consulting room, I scrolled quickly through her record. I spotted the problem straight away: the CCG had blocked the prescription of her medication due to rising costs. They insisted it was almost identical to Sudafed and that she should just use that instead.

I sympathised with Diane, then wrote to the CCG asking for special dispensation. She had trialled so many different medications, including Sudafed, which had not worked at all. She had been on an expensive journey through specialists on the NHS, so surely it was better to keep her on her existing medication as it worked so well.

But the CCG wanted a consultant to demonstrate its efficacy. Unfortunately, the consultant who had painstakingly supported Diane over the years had now retired. I had letters of recommendation, but the CCG wanted a new letter detailing its precise benefits over other treatments. I argued that the most valuable evidence was the patient's experience, as documented. I was informed that it was not their policy to accept this as adequate justification.

We kept fighting and, in the meantime, Diane tried a range of different decongestants, cough suppressant medicines and nasal sprays. She remained one of those difficult cases. Nothing else worked. We tried acupuncture and herbal remedies. All the while, she coughed and coughed.

Her mood started to drop, and she stopped entertaining. She gave up her talks. As she became a little less herself each time I saw her, robbed of her enjoyment of life by her illness, my concern for her increased.

At least her situation wasn't gravely serious. There must surely be a way to help her live to the full, and I was determined to go on looking for it.

*

The next time I saw Diane, she looked upset. She told me that her constant coughing was causing a prolapse. Every time she coughed, she could feel something bulging out through her vagina. She had not had children, which made this condition unusual. Most commonly, a prolapsed womb comes from weakening of the pelvic floor after the vaginal delivery of babies. However, a very prolonged cough like hers could certainly raise intra-abdominal pressure and contribute to a uterine prolapse, so I examined her.

Sure enough, a smooth, pink, grapefruit-like protrusion could be seen appearing down through the dark vaginal cave when she coughed. Her womb also felt bulky. We organised an ultrasound and referred her to the Urogynaecology Team. This is the team who specialise in repair of vaginal and uterine prolapse, and the strengthening of the pelvic floor.

Her ultrasound came back showing fibroids. This is unusual but not unheard of in someone in their late fifties or sixties. Now we waited for the urogynaecology appointment to come through.

Two months later, Diane appeared on my morning list. I opened the door and called her in. She pushed past me into the room and sat on the chair glaring up at me.

'Have you completely lost your mind?' she snapped, her head twitching backwards and forwards with pent-up energy. 'Why on earth did you send me to a clap clinic?'

I was bewildered. 'Ummm...'

'Yes, yes!' she shouted. 'Ummm away! I arrived at my appointment yesterday expecting to see a gynaecologist and have a discussion about a hysterectomy or something. But *no*, I sat down and this boy – this *boy!* – asking me about how many times I have had sex in the last six months and with whom. Well, I haven't had sex for thirty-five years, and I told him so in no uncertain terms. He then asks me why I have come to a Sexual Health Clinic if I haven't had sex.'

She paused to take a large in-breath before proceeding.

'And so, Dr Marshall-Andrews, I ask you again: have you completely lost your mind?'

My heart sank. I knew exactly what had happened. The Referral Management Service, in its great wisdom, had redirected my referral of Diane to the Sexual Health Clinic.

The Referral Management Service is supposed to save money. It ensures that only relevant referrals make it through to the hospital. When it was founded, all referrals coming from GPs were screened by other GPs, judged against a plethora of policies, then either passed on to an administrator, who would call the patient and discuss which hospital they would like to go to, or rejected and sent back to the GP. Initially this was quite helpful. GPs couldn't possibly be expected to know all the possible and rapidly increasing number of services that might be available, and patients got to choose where and when they were seen.

However, over time and under successive governments, funding for the Referral Management Service dwindled. It could no longer afford to pay GPs to screen the referrals, or to employ people to take the time to speak to patients about where they wanted to go. So now the service is run by non-medical staff following strict protocols. Patients are simply allocated the next appointment that comes up somewhere near them. Sometimes it's not even that near.

In theory this should all still work – but it doesn't. A lot of referrals are hard to fit into a protocol. Patients sometimes present with unusual complaints or have unusual circumstances. Much of the time, the admin team members make mistakes because they don't fully understand the referral. And why should they? They are not doctors. Recently, a patient in a wheelchair burst into my room asking me why I had referred him all the way to Epsom for his orthopaedic review when he only had one leg.

I apologised profusely to Diane and promised I would talk to the 'service' and get her seen in a more appropriate place as soon as possible. We'd lost a bit of time in getting to the root of her problems, that was all. Then, as she was leaving, she turned round to me and said, 'Just so you know – I have started bleeding down there. A *lot*.'

This was worrying. But actually, it made things easier, as now I could tick a box on the 'two-week rule' pathway. This is a pathway made for referrals where there is a suspicion of cancer. Thankfully, two-week-rule referrals do not go through the Referral Management Service – yet.

Ten days later I had a letter back from the gynaecologists. They had seen Diane, and reassured her that in spite of the bleeding, her problem was just fibroids. Still, they wanted to do a hysteroscopy (a camera into the womb) just in case.

*

The next time she came back to see me, Diane's story had taken a suddenly far darker turn. Her suspected fibroids had been further investigated with a biopsy. The biopsy found a rare form of cancer called a leiomyosarcoma. This can be aggressive, they had told her.

Diane and I sat there together as she pivoted between the end of one chapter of her life and the beginning of the last.

People confront death in a multitude of different ways. Diane faced hers with a high level of efficiency and organisation. As with everything, there were pros and cons to this strategy.

If cancers have characters, then a leiomyosarcoma of the uterus is a rogue Royal Marine. It is rare and aggressive, but cunning. It lies camouflaged and waits. It strategically deploys its resources around the battleground of the body and then it relentlessly attacks. Diane underwent brutal radiotherapy and chemotherapy, which bought her a year or so, but damaged her gut and hair and skin. Her thinness became more pronounced, and her twitchy bird-like energy faded.

Even so, she embarked on a desperate race to categorise, order and despatch her vast collection of African artefacts. She drew up complex systems of organisation depending on age, place of origin, value, and which of her friends liked the item best.

She scheduled a complete overhaul of the two-storey flat, funded by complex financing processes. As her health started to fail her, these ambitious plans became more and more unachievable. But living in many remote areas of the world had given her a grim determination, which showed itself now. Relentlessly she ploughed on, with true grit.

Towards the end of her life, I popped in to see her. It was a Saturday morning and my children were all busy, so I had some time. I was glad of it.

She buzzed me into her flat. She was standing in her long white nightie. It had white embroidery around the neck and cuffs, but from the waist down it was dark red with blood and clung like static to her thin legs. She was holding a clipboard with long lists and tables of numbers on it. Her bony arms protruded from the elbow-length sleeves and her hair had become completely wild and upstanding on her head. She looked like a frightened bird that had been shot out of the sky.

There were trails of blood all around the flat, but mostly in the bedroom, which was the designated the epicentre, the headquarters, of the sorting process. There was a lot of blood on the bed sheets. Diane was moving around the flat, unsteadily making crosses and adding numbers to the lists on her clipboard.

Clothes, wooden figures, bowls, books and jewellery were stacked in neat piles with labels over every surface. Some of the piles had been knocked over and lay in bloody puddles on the floor.

I followed her around for a bit while she jabbed her finger at different items, asking me to read out the number on the Post-it note that had been stuck on it.

'Would you like this?' she asked, holding out a small pottery bowl, with a Post-it note with the number '34c' scrawled on it. She told me she had acquired it in Gabon.

'Diane, I think you are bleeding,' I said.

She looked down at the dark red patch on her nightie and then back up at me. Her eyes widened as if she had only just noticed.

'Is this it? Am I dying right now?' she asked, and she broke down in tears. 'I haven't finished the patio! I wanted a Moroccan feel.'

I sat down next to her and held her thin body while she cried and cried. We slowly made our way to the bathroom, which was in the middle of being turned into a Turkish hammam. She got in the bath while I changed her bed sheets and tried to get rid of as much blood from the floor as possible. My husband will tell you that I have a rather haphazard approach to cleaning, but by the time she came out of the bathroom, the flat at least looked less like a teen horror film.

I called the Palliative Care Team. They were incredible, as they usually are. They would send someone over straight away, and try to admit her to the hospice later today or tomorrow. I sat with Diane until they arrived. As the adrenalin levels calmed in her body, she grew weaker and got into bed. She looked terribly pale and drifted in and out of sleep. Even in her half-consciousness, with her eyes closed, she managed to give me directions about items of clothing that needed to be moved from pile to pile. Her friends kept changing their minds about the things they wanted. People are so fickle nowadays.

The Palliative Care Team arrived. White knights to the rescue. Diane refused to go initially. She still had too much to do. We managed to persuade her to go into the hospice to help with the bleeding. As they left the flat, I caught a glimpse of the builders arriving to work on the Moroccan patio. Diane died a few days later. I have the tiny pottery bowl she left me on my desk. It still has the Post-it note with '34c' scrawled on it.

Diane never asked me if her misguided referral by the Referral Management Service had cost her her life. The system had certainly let her down. But had ending up in the Sexual Health Clinic instead of the gynaecology clinic been pivotal to her survival? I think we both wondered if it had. If she had seen the urogynaecologist I had referred her to three months earlier, would her prognosis have been different?

It's possible. It was a system error. In spite of all our technological advances, sending a referral through the current system is akin to sending a carrier pigeon. Instead of dodging hawks and bad weather, today's electronic messages must dodge the obstacles of misinterpretation, redirection, rejection and technical error. Having a fully qualified professional in place to sort through referrals may be more expensive up front, but it will save money, and lives, further down the line.

In the end, Diane died peacefully. Her flat was sold. I hope the new owners enjoyed the Moroccan patio and hammam-style bathroom. It's impossible to say whether an earlier diagnosis would have changed the course of her illness dramatically – but it's a question I still hold.

*

But sometimes it isn't just the system that fails – people do. Doctors are human beings. What that means is that doctors will sometimes make mistakes. We need to accept that medical error will happen. It is inevitable.

When it does, we need a robust structure that responds both effectively and compassionately. It needs to do two things: to help patients move forward with their lives, and to enable doctors to learn so that the mistake, whatever it was, will not be repeated.

Medical error is one of the biggest fears of any doctor or patient. There are two reasons why. First and foremost, we deal daily with suffering, pain and illness. We know that the decisions we make can lead to happiness and a cure, or disability and death. Error understandably haunts us, for no one wants to inflict pain or exacerbate another person's suffering.

The second reason is the prospect of courts, disciplinary hearings and compensation payments. These are the fears that lead to defensive medicine. They also hinder investigation and block the opportunity for a really important kind of learning: learning through error.

Many years ago, I met Tozar. Tozar was a fifty-three-year-old man who loved to cycle. He rode his bike for hours every weekend. His favourite route was up over the Sussex Downs. He would go early in the morning; he loved the pregnant stillness of the air before the sun climbed higher in the sky. This was the time of day that belonged to the birds and the odd rabbit dashing into the hedgerows. Sometimes he would see a late fox trotting back to its den.

One Sunday morning, he was flying along the homeward road thinking of the breakfast his wife would make him: a Sunday omelette with cheese and chillies and possibly tomatoes. He would put his bike away, shower and settle himself at his table in eager anticipation of his well-earned reward. But as he pelted down the road that snakes off Ditchling Beacon, his tyre slipped and the bike careered out of control. In that moment, he saw the flash of the bonnet of a car speeding up the hill towards him. With superhuman strength, he managed to wrench the handlebars back towards the verge and he and his bike flew into the ditch, narrowly avoiding the Mini Cooper racing past.

He lay in the ditch, wheels and mind spinning for several minutes. Slowly he began assessing the damage to himself and his beloved bike. He could move his legs and arms and his bike was amazingly unscathed. Shakily he managed to get the rest of the way home, but during the afternoon his upper abdomen became sore and tender and painful when touched.

First thing on Monday morning, he was sitting in my clinic describing the events of the previous day. I examined his abdomen and found that there was no rigid guarding of the muscles or masses. His chest was clear and breathing was unrestricted. I advised painkillers and to come back if his symptoms were not improving.

About three months later on a wintery afternoon before surgery, my colleague Francis came in to see me. He smiled a half-smile in response to my cheery greeting. There was a slight tremor in the hand he laid on my shoulder, and he fixed his eyes on me. I realised that he was about to deliver bad news. I felt my heart rate pick up and my body temperature rise. I struggled to concentrate on what he was saying.

Tozar had come to see him. He looked pale and his abdominal pain had worsened. By the time he saw Francis he was very anaemic and his abdomen was tender and distended. I had missed a stomach ulcer, which was now causing internal bleeding.

Here it was, my first big error.

I felt sick, brain spinning, heart pounding. I tried to focus on Francis's voice. Tozar had made a complaint, and I needed to call my Medical Defence Union. I nodded dumbly. Francis patted me on the back.

'Don't worry,' he said. 'It happens to the best of us.'

I went to the toilet and cried. After my surgery ended, I called the MDU. They advised me to write my response, detailing my position and justification. 'Don't do anything without talking to us first,' was their clear guidance. 'Don't admit anything and don't speak or write to the patient without our advice,' they said to me. But I desperately wanted to call Tozar. I wanted to apologise to him.

My overriding feeling was guilt. I felt so sorry that I had delayed his diagnosis and that this might affect the outcome of his illness. I called friends in the medical profession, but they all gave me the same advice as the MDU.

'Laura, you are a professional. You gave your advice to the best of your ability. Let the lawyers handle it. Don't admit culpability or apologise. Do everything in writing and do it through your defence union.'

The next day, I went into the practice to see Francis.

'How is Tozar?' I asked.

'He is seeing the gastroenterologist tomorrow. He is angry but he's okay. I can look after him from now on. Try not to worry.'

All through my morning clinic, I couldn't shake off an awful, heavy feeling in the pit of my stomach. At midday, I sat at my desk reading through Tozar's notes, wishing I could turn back the clock and make a different plan. I would ask him to come back in two weeks if his abdomen was still sore. He would have come back and then I would have realised that the issue wasn't a muscle injury, and I would have referred him on.

But something else needed to come first. I reached over and dialled Tozar's number. I knew clearly that I needed to talk to him. I needed to apologise. It might be the end of my career and it would certainly be a very uncomfortable experience, but I knew it was the right thing to do, for him and for me.

He answered the phone. I took a deep breath.

'Hi – is that Tozar? It's Dr Laura Marshall-Andrews here.'

'Oh. Hello.' There was a pause. He sounded taken aback.

'I just wanted to call to apologise,' I ploughed on. 'I know that won't make things better for you, but I just wanted you to know that I am sorry. I want you to know that I won't forget the lessons I have learnt from this.'

We sat in silence for a few long seconds. I realised I had tears running down my face, but I tried to keep my voice steady.

'Good luck tomorrow with the gastroenterologist,' I managed to say.

'You really should have brought me back to check that pain and not just assumed it was a muscle injury,' he replied.

'I know. I am sorry.' I paused again.

'Thank you for phoning.' His voice softened a bit. 'That must have been hard.' He put the receiver down. I sat staring at the phone, wondering what would happen next.

About six weeks later, I saw Tozar's name on my morning surgery list. He came into my room and told me about the gastroenterologist's appointment and his prognosis, which was good. He'd had surgery and developed a rash on his leg. I gave him some cream and he left. He saw me several times after that and we never mentioned our telephone conversation. He must have dropped the complaint. I didn't hear anything more about it.

I often tell this story to my trainees and medical students. It is a good lesson in the diagnosis of a peptic ulcer and the concept of 'early anchoring', a cognitive bias in medical practice where the doctor can fix too early on the first diagnosis that seems to make sense. It is also a lesson in the kindness and forgiveness of patients. I remember Tozar with affection, and find myself thinking of him often. Fortunately he did well with the treatment and was still cycling on the Downs last time I saw him. It could have been a different story; at the time that he forgave me he did not know what the outcome would be. Still, he was prepared to let go of what had happened.

But I am very much aware that the system doesn't easily allow patients to let go. Often it needs blame and accusation. Without those things, it has no way to recompense those who have suffered.

*

Early in my career, I was a junior doctor for six months on the obstetrics and gynaecology wards at Chelsea and Westminster Hospital. I had some of the most inspiring and also some of the most traumatic experiences of my career over these months.

'Obs and gynae' is one of the specialties that suffers most litigation. Childbirth is an intrinsically dangerous time for both the mother and the baby. In countries without well-funded healthcare systems, it is still the biggest killer of women and infants.

The major breakthrough in saving maternal and perinatal life has been the lower-segment caesarean section, which has transformed childbirth into a much safer process. As operations go, it is relatively simple and low-risk. A low incision is made above the mother's pubic bone into the uterus and the baby is extracted without having to pass through the ridiculously narrow birth canal. It is a very safe procedure and represents a 'get out of jail free card' for difficult, obstructed labours.

I often observed a tension in delivery rooms between the midwife and the obstetric surgeon. Midwives tended to encourage vaginal deliveries – they 'back the woman' to 'do it herself', as most women want to. The surgeon, however, sees the possible complications looming and usually advises surgery at a lower threshold.

The most common danger sign in labour is 'foetal distress'. This is picked up by changes in the baby's heart rate during and after uterine contractions. It is a sign that the baby is losing oxygen to the brain, and it usually means that a caesarean section is required to prevent the baby from sustaining lasting brain damage. Usually, patients are happy to be guided by the teams advising them. But not always.

When I was a junior on the obs and gynae ward, a dark story hung over the department. Two years previously, a mother came onto the ward with her partner. She was in established labour and had been very keen to deliver her first child at home. Halfway through the labour, the midwife had persuaded her to come into hospital as the baby's heart rate was not picking up well after each contraction. It is normal for a baby's heart rate to slow during a contraction, but it usually speeds up again as the uterus relaxes. If the heart rate does not accelerate after the contraction, there may be a problem; for example, the umbilical cord, which connects the baby to the mother, may be looped around the baby's neck, constricting blood flow to the baby and particularly to the brain. If this persists, the baby needs to be delivered by caesarean section as an emergency. Most mothers and babies will then be completely well.

But this mother did not want to deliver in this way. She was adamant that the best thing for her and the baby was a vaginal delivery. The surgeon on duty at the time was a tall, rather stern woman. She was clear with the mother that she was very concerned about the baby and that she was keen to operate as soon as possible. The surgeon documented their conversation carefully. But the mother still refused.

As time went on, the baby's heart rate took longer and longer to recover after each contraction. Three times, the surgeon went back to try to persuade her to consent to a lower-segment caesarean section. Each time, she meticulously documented the conversation. The surgeon also called her consultant and the paediatric consultant. All three doctors tried to talk to the mother and father, in vain. Unless they operated immediately, they told them (and possibly by this stage, even if they did), their baby would have permanent brain damage. The midwife also wanted the caesarean by now, and she too explained the potential consequences of not operating.

But the mother remained adamant – she would not consent. She insisted on proceeding with vaginal delivery. In her view, it was the right and natural thing – and that was what she wanted. It would turn out, years down the line, that the mother had been very suspicious of doctors and did not trust them. She was terrified after having heard and believed tales of them operating for fun on women in labour. Despite the surgeon's and the consultants' repeated pleas, she refused to undergo an LSCS.

By now the baby's heart rate had slowed right down. When she was eventually born, she was barely alive. The paediatricians spent most of the night resuscitating her, but she suffered extreme damage to her brain, resulting in very severe cerebral palsy.

While I was working on the ward, there was an ongoing court case resulting from all this. The mother and father sued the surgeon for not explaining the situation clearly to them. They alleged that they had not been made aware of the seriousness of the situation, and the consequences of the different courses of action. They had to file that lawsuit in order to get financial compensation to look after their disabled child. They had to prove negligence. This was a lengthy and distressing process for all parties involved.

Despite the surgeon's detailed notes, and the substantiating evidence of the midwife and consultants, the court ruled in favour of the parents. They would get their compensation. The surgeon left medicine.

This story is a tragedy in every way. A baby was injured, and a good doctor lost her job. It was deeply damaging to everyone involved, and any important lessons we could have learnt were lost in recrimination and rebuke. Events like this affect the whole culture of the medical profession. They turn patient and doctor into adversaries. It doesn't have to be like this.

In a system that doesn't need to apportion blame, the mother and father could have received a standard compensation for their baby's preventable injury without having to fight a vicious court case. Then, in a separate inquiry, the events of that afternoon could have been examined. Was there any way that communication between doctor and patient could have been handled differently? Is there anything we can all learn? How can we try to prevent it from happening again?

It is impossible for a doctor and a patient to work well together if they do not trust each other. If the patient fears the doctor might intentionally harm them, they will clearly struggle to engage in the process wholeheartedly. Likewise, if the doctor fears the patient they are treating might turn into an adversary and sue them or prosecute them, they too will struggle to engage openly. Our current system of litigation and compensation sets us in opposition to our patients. We must find ways to allow investigation of procedures and actions, without the doctor or other medical practitioner being thrust into the dock and accused.

Back then, as a bright-eyed, enthusiastic young medical student, I had no way of knowing that one day I would be the doctor standing in that dock.

*

Angie was a big woman. She approached six foot with bare feet, which was how she sometimes attended the surgery. Her heavy, dark features could once have been considered beautiful, but loose flesh now fell around her jowls and her mouth was fixed in a permanent downturn. She cut a dark, menacing figure as he glared down at Gaynor. Gaynor was kind-hearted and brave. She had had her fair share of violence in her life and was well used to facing up to angry people.

'Oh, for fuck's sake!' Angie was shouting as I came up the stairs. 'Give me my fucking medication, you stupid woman!'

Her medication was a strong opiate drug called oxycodone. Angie was dealing with chronic pain, which lay between her groin and her anus in an area called the perineum. It is a smooth area with a few organs close by which could have caused the pain. She had been seen by gynaecologists and urologists, who specialise in the female pelvic anatomy, but they could not find any cause. Then she'd been referred to the pain clinic, which was how she had got started on oxycodone. It worked initially, and then she had simply become addicted to it. An opiate drug that had started off as a solution ended up a big part of her problems.

We had been trying to help her come off her prescription by looking for the root of the physical pain that had made her seek out such an addictive drug in the first place. We had referred her for counselling and encouraged her to join singing groups and art classes. Throughout all of our investigations, however, the shadow of Angie's difficult past had hovered in the background like a dark spectre that could not be engaged with. I sensed that a great deal of her story was untold; there was certainly a deep well of unaddressed anger inside her and it easily spilled over.

Gaynor also understood this. She didn't seem too fazed by all the shouting. She was trying to explain to Angie that the system was showing she had had her weekly allowance of oxycodone already, and that she wasn't due more for another four days.

'Well – I never picked that up,' she was screaming. 'Someone else must have got it.'

Gaynor went on talking to her gently, trying to ascertain what had happened to the prescription. She obviously knew she had collected it herself.

'Okay, Angie, I am so sorry about that,' she said. 'We'll call the chemist and see if they remember who collected it.'

'Oh, for fuck's sake!' she shouted again. 'Don't you believe me? I am not standing for this. I'm calling my lawyer.' She strode over to me and pushed her face up against mine. 'You better get ready,' she said menacingly. Then she shoved me out of the way and stormed out of the door.

'Bye, Angie,' I called after her. She flicked me a finger as she disappeared off down the road. A day or so later, she was back. Her attempts to get extra prescriptions became a regular occurrence. They never succeeded. No doctor would have agreed to what she was asking. It would endanger her life.

And then one day when she came to see me, she told me that she wanted four months of medication in one go. This sounded like madness. I refused straight away. She threatened to take me to court, but it was an empty threat. She was like a child, raging against the world. She lied a lot, in keeping with her illness. But I knew that this wasn't really her – she was in the grip of a powerful force determining her behaviour.

This time, though, she was certainly extra-persistent. Stumbling over her words, she tried to explain that she had a special, *different* reason for asking.

'Okay, Angie,' I said eventually, 'tell me why you think I should give you this medication.' She told me that an old acquaintance had made her an offer that could give her the chance to get away from all her problems – maybe even to make a fresh start.

'Come on, doc, please – this is my only way out. I've got to get out of that stinking hole or I'll die there.'

Angie meant her tiny basement flat, where damp leaked permanently down the back wall of the small kitchenette. Living there, the only thing she had to look forward to was the dose of oxycodone she took every six hours. Her life hadn't always been like this. When she was in her late teens she had travelled all over the world, working for English-speaking travel-guide outlets wherever she went as a way of funding her wanderlust. It had kept her happy for a long time – until she was forced to come back to the UK and her life nosedived into the tiny dark space that she now inhabited.

An old acquaintance she had spent some time with when she was on her travels had recently set up a new adventure-guide company in Peru and had asked her to join him out there. This friend was willing to take a chance on Angie, for old times' sake. Angie would fly to Peru and join her friend in the Andes. They would then spend four months leading a group of tourists around the little-known paths, forgotten mountain passes and villages that had been frequented by the Inca.

At first, I didn't believe this was the reason Angie was asking for her drugs in such a large quantity. I figured, like the doctors before me, that she wanted to either sell it or take larger quantities of it than we were eking out to her.

'But this is my big break, doc,' she pleaded. 'I'm never gonna get better living in that shit-hole with all those crackheads around me.'

I had to agree that her prospects seemed grim. It was understandable that she felt little hope or motivation for the future. It niggled at me. By not prescribing the medication as she wanted, was I preventing her from a chance at a new life? I spoke to my Medical Defence Union who told me to use my clinical judgment. If there was a complaint, they would help me, but it was up to me to make the decision.

I spoke to several other GPs who all said I was mad to even consider what Angie was asking. Doctors have an interesting perception of risk. When debating a difficult, risk-filled decision with a patient, we often perceive the risk as our own. I suppose in a sense there is danger to our professional integrity. However, it seemed to me that the real risk was being taken by the patient. It is their life to live and they who will live or die as a consequence of their decisions.

'If you give her what she wants and she overdoses and dies from oxycodone – or gets injured in the middle of nowhere – then you are liable, Laura!' said a medical friend anxiously. 'I understand – you want to give this lady a chance. But it's too big a risk. If this goes wrong, you'll lose your licence.'

Here again was the familiar caution of our profession. However, in my opinion, we were already giving her weekly amounts of medication, which were probably enough to kill her if she took it all at once. She never had. I did not think she was suicidal. Essentially, it came down to trust. Did I trust that she was capable enough to manage her medication on the road and not put herself or anyone else at risk of harm? The benefit to her was great – this could potentially change her life forever. It really could be the chance of a new beginning, not only because it would catapult her out of her miserable existence, but also because if I showed that I trusted her, then it gave her a sense of value and worth.

I spoke to the substance misuse team. Their advice was not to give her the oxycodone. However, when I talked one-to-one with the lead doctor there, he agreed that it was a tough call and that, in reality, the risk of Angie harming herself was low and the chance of potential gain was high. He would not condone it formally, but I felt it was the fear of losing his job that was stopping him, rather than a fear for the patient's wellbeing or safety.

Angie came in to see me again. She was desperate for this trip to happen. She felt it was her one big break that could spike her out of the trap she was currently in.

'Angie, I am minded to try to help you with this. But I need you to prove your commitment and I need to know that the offer and the job are real,' I said to her.

She sat looking at me. For once she was not threatening me with violence or legal action. 'All right,' she said. Later that day she brought a printed email trail from the friend's travel agency. I called the head guy, who confirmed it. They would agree to fund Angie's trip if I was happy that she was safe to go.

We had three weeks before she left. The process of getting off a drug like oxycodone has to be managed very carefully. We agreed that she would reduce her dose from 5mg four times a day, to 5mg twice a day. I would then give her enough to reduce again, to 2.5mg of oxycodone, once a day, over the next five weeks while she was leading the trek in the Andes. She should be safe to stop completely then.

Four days before she left, she came to see me. She had managed to get down to 5mg twice a day. Everything seemed to be in order. However, I was still about to give a massive quantity of highly addictive medication to a woman with a history of violence and allow her to take it away for four months.

'Angie, my job and your life are riding on you now. You know that, don't you?'

She scowled heavily.

'What do you want, a fucking medal?' she sounded aggressive, but I was used to that. I thought that underneath, she probably did appreciate the chance I was taking. This was a chance to take her life in a new and much more positive direction – and as such, it was all a bit overwhelming for her. She didn't know how to express that kind of emotion.

'No, Angie.' I gave her a smile. 'I was thinking more... chocolates, flowers, thank you – that sort of thing.'

'Whatever,' she said. She picked up the prescription and walked out.

The next day, our receptionist Rachel called me up. Angie was in Reception and refusing to leave until she had seen me. My heart started pounding as I walked up the stairs. 'Please don't let her have "lost" the prescription,' I prayed. I steeled myself for a confrontation.

She walked up to me as I entered the waiting room – and abruptly thrust a Crunchie bar into my hand. Not quite a box of Milk Tray, but I was suddenly quite touched. For just a moment, she looked me in the eye.

'Thank you,' she said gruffly. Then she turned on her heel and left.

That was the last time I saw her.

We got a call from a hospital somewhere in the Andes just under five months later saying that Angie had come to them for help with the final stages of her withdrawal from oxycodone. She had made the prescription last longer than we'd initially intended by coming down faster to start with, then eking the last 2.5mg tablets out at the end. They wanted to check out her story.

Although that Crunchie was the only thanks I ever got, I knew I'd made a difference to Angie's life. I'd believed in her, and been prepared to take a chance.

Two years later, Angie came back into the practice. She wanted to register with us again. She was tanned, our receptionist said, and looked well. But by now, she had moved to a bigger house outside our catchment area. Her life really did seem to have improved. Rachel gave her the number of a practice nearer her new address.

I was delighted to hear how much better she was doing and wondered if there might be a message for me – something to show that she remembered the chance I'd taken on her. I asked our receptionist.

'Oh yes. She said to say hi,' she replied.

'Nothing else?'

'No, just hi.'

Ah, well. Perhaps that Crunchie said it all.

*

'Laura – you've got Connor booked to see you this morning,' Gaynor warned me. 'Just thought you'd appreciate the heads-up.'

I certainly did. All the practice staff knew Connor, and everybody liked him. But being well known to staff at a practice is not a good sign. It usually means you are very ill, or very annoying. Connor was very ill. He had teetered on the edge of dying for many years. A consultation with him would always need careful preparation.

Connor was a deeply troubled man who had serious unresolved issues. His list of medications was longer than my forearm: for heart and kidney failure, to suppress his out-of-control immune system and to support his kidney transplant. And then there were the medications to treat the side effects of his other medications. He'd been a patient at the practice long before I arrived. A funny and sociable man, he'd once lived life hard despite his significant illnesses, and formed the centre of a fun-loving crowd. But over the years, he had gradually lost much of his humour as his illnesses wore him down. 'Better make the most of it, doc,' was one of his favourite expressions. He'd always lived like he might die tomorrow, and it was now a real and constant possibility. He'd always liked a drink – whisky was his tipple, as it had been his mother's. He smoked forty cigarettes a day.

His most serious problem was his Crohn's disease, an autoimmune condition, which tends to flare up in a patient's twenties. Among other things, it causes deep fissuring ulcers through the bowel which result in pain and bleeding. If not treated, Crohn's can lead to perforation of the bowel and death. The reason behind autoimmune diseases such as Crohn's developing is a bit of a mystery. It is likely to be due to a mesh of factors, some genetic and others environmental. Perhaps a viral illness stimulates the production of particular antibodies that unfortunately also attack the bowel. Perhaps excessive cleanliness during childhood prevents normal development of the immune system. Perhaps it is triggered by periods of intense stress and poor diet. The honest truth is – we don't really know what triggers it, or why people suffer from this devastating disease.

Nowadays, Crohn's can be relatively well treated with a combination of diet, exercise, stress management, surgery and immunosuppressant medication. But this medication brings its own complications, and Connor unfortunately suffered most of them. His kidney failure and heart failure resulted from these treatments and had led to his transplant. He was constantly in hospital.

His biggest complaint, one which permeated every aspect of his life, was the constant pain he was in as a result of his Crohn's. His was a deep, searing, debilitating abdominal pain. But no one really knew the exact cause. He had very little bowel left, and he had been extensively imaged without finding any conclusive cause of his intense discomfort. We tried everything: nerve-blocking injections, antidepressants, multiple different pain medications and counselling.

While recovering from one of his extensive operations, he was started on fentanyl, the opiate medication I had seen patients like Jasper becoming addicted to. He was given this in the form of lollipops, which the patient sucks for a quick release of strong pain relief. These lollipops are used post-operatively when patients need fast-acting analgesia before being turned over, or if they're having painful dressings or procedures. They are expensive.

By the time I met Connor, he was addicted to fentanyl lollies. They were the only thing that took away his pain. Even fentanyl in other formats didn't seem to work – not tablets, not patches, not injections. Connor's life expectancy was limited. All other pain relief had failed. So we decided to continue with his fentanyl lollipop prescription. It was well controlled and issued to him on a fortnightly basis.

Then his mother became very ill. For several months he travelled back and forth to their home near Manchester to visit her, which greatly increased his pain.

I thought Connor's pain was most likely a combination of emotional distress deeply buried in his body, caused by both his extensive operations and disease processes and by his emotional turmoil. The distress of his mother's impending death combined with long hours sitting cramped and uncomfortable on trains and carrying heavy bags was making him thoroughly miserable. She then died, and Connor, already struggling with poor health, was plunged into grief.

While all this was going on, the Medicines Management Team had noticed the cost of his prescription. They grew steadily more aggressive in their communications about it. They wanted Connor off fentanyl lollipops. They suggested using other forms of fentanyl we had already tried – anything to get him off this most expensive form of the drug. But I did not agree with the MMT. I believed that what Connor was experiencing had complex causes. These causes ranged from the physical changes resulting from his surgery and the trauma of serious disease, to the death of his mother and other shadowy events in his childhood. Until we could unpick and help treat these underpinning causes of his pain, he would remain addicted to this soothing and sedating medicine.

Opiates are a horrible class of drug. They ruin lives. I never prescribe them to patients with long-term pain, but it was hard to see how stopping them was going to help Connor. It felt cruel to end the treatment without being able to offer him an effective alternative.

I was therefore not prepared to stop his prescription.

Once again, I met with Rachel from the MMT. This time, though, the meeting was more difficult than it had been when we clashed over Karen and her need for Armour Thyroid. It was harder to prove an economic case for Connor. His fentanyl lollipops did not enable him to work or contribute to society, they just made his desperate life more bearable. The meeting ended inconclusively. I was unsure what was going to happen next. I could only hope that the matter would be left there.

But it wasn't. A few weeks later, an email arrived. I had been summoned to appear before the Performers' Advisory Group. At first, I wasn't sure exactly what this meant. But as I read and re-read the email, I realised I had been reported to this disciplinary body by the MMT.

The PAG is a disciplinary panel run by NHS England. It has the power to remove a doctor's licence to practice in the NHS. The panel date was set for three months' time, in the middle of January.

I have known of doctors who have attempted suicide, sometimes successfully, in the face of professional investigations. It is certainly no picnic. For me, I was sure of one thing. If I couldn't do what I believed was right for my patients, then I did not want to be a doctor.

The summons played on my mind through the rest of the day, sending shocks of adrenalin and cold sweats across my body. I tried to concentrate on my work, on my patients and their problems, but it kept slipping back into my consciousness. I could not face the humiliation and I was still unclear exactly what the charges against me were. But later on that evening, I breathed slowly and, keeping as calm as I was able to, I read the whole email with great care. It cited concerns over the practice's prescribing of opiate medication (the class of medicine fentanyl belongs to). No reference was made to the efforts we had put into reducing these medications for many of our patients.

At the next practice meeting one lunch time, I revealed my situation to the team. There was an overwhelming sense of shock. We had tried so hard to do the right thing for our patients: to listen to them, to act in ways which had their best interests at heart, to reduce medication use and to prescribe with wisdom and care.

'They've got it in for you, Laura. They always have had,' said Nick, one of my newly qualified GPs who also did some part-time work at the CCG.

'I've heard them talking about you,' he went on. 'They don't like people doing things differently. It scares them – makes them think they are losing control.'

A few weeks later, another email arrived from the CCG. It told me that the case against me was widening. Now, they informed me, there were concerns about the practice's prescription of controlled drugs, my approach to prescribing unlicensed medication, my engagement with prescribing colleagues in the Clinical Commissioning Group, and the implications of this on my contractual agreement as a GP. That meant my ability to work within the NHS.

Underneath all this was a list of counsellors and support groups and the suggestion that I might want to 'inform my defence union'. The email helpfully concluded: 'We understand this can be a very stressful time.'

When I told Gary all of this, he was absolutely incandescent with rage.

'How dare they do this to us, to you?' he stormed. 'Petty and narrow-minded, that's what they are.'

'Don't let it get to you, Laura,' said Lolita Simcock when I showed her the emails. 'You don't need counsellors – you've got us. We are all behind you – what we've done here is incredible. They are just jealous.'

So over the next few months, we worked together on our defence. I wrote up the histories of Karen and Connor in more detail, with the evidence behind our decision-making. The whole team helped to put together a compelling case.

Several weeks before the day of the 'trial', I received another email from the doctor leading the investigation at the PAG. He asked that information around the allegations be sent to him.

I sent him the files we had created and, as an aside, I asked if he could send me the final list of exactly what the charges against me were. He seemed surprised that I had not already been sent this, and forwarded me a pack of documents. I sat at the computer at our makeshift desk in the bedroom to read it that evening. As the document opened on the screen in front of me, I realised that the list was shockingly long.

Slowly I read through the sheet. The main cases were as we had suspected: Connor and Karen – but they didn't stop there. The PAG had really gone to town. It was clear from the long list of suggested General Medical Council violations that somebody was gunning for the removal of my licence to practise medicine.

GMC 18 – FAILURE TO MAKE GOOD USE OF THE RESOURCES AVAILABLE TO YOU

GMC 22 – FAILURE TO TAKE PART IN SYSTEMS OF QUALITY ASSURANCE

GMC 35 – FAILURE TO WORK COLLABORATIVELY WITH COLLEAGUES

GMC 37 – FAILURE TO BE AWARE OF HOW YOUR BEHAVIOUR MAY INFLUENCE OTHERS WITHIN THE TEAM

GMC 11 – FAILURE TO TAKE ACCOUNT OF CLINICAL GUIDELINES

GMC 69 – FAILURE TO HAVE THE SUFFICIENT EXPERIENCE OR EXPERTISE TO PRESCRIBE UNLICENSED MEDICATION

GMC 2d – FAILURE TO DEMONSTRATE EFFECTIVE TEAM WORKING AND LEADERSHIP

GMC 2g – FAILURE TO USE RESOURCES EFFECTIVELY FOR THE BENEFIT OF PATIENTS AND THE PUBLIC

GMC 4 – FAILURE TO WORK WITH OTHER PEOPLE AND TEAMS TO MAINTAIN AND IMPROVE PERFORMANCE

GMC 79 – FAILURE TO DEMONSTRATE LEADERSHIP IN MANAGING AND USING RECOURSE EFFECTIVELY, INCLUDING THE ALLOCATION AND SETTING OF PRIORITIES WITHIN YOUR ORGANISATION

GMC 84 – FAILURE TO SHOW THAT TAKING CARE OF PATIENTS IS YOUR FIRST CONCERN AND TO WORK WITHIN YOUR RESOURCES

GMC 85 – FAILURE TO PROVIDE THE BEST POSSIBLE SERVICE TO YOUR PATIENTS WITHIN YOUR CAPACITY AND RESOURCE.

GMC 16 – FAILURE TO PROVIDE THE BEST EFFECTIVE TREATMENT BASED ON THE BEST EVIDENCE AVAILABLE

I sat there staring. None of this was true. These charges felt to me like the hurt pride of a few individuals. They also felt vindictive.

Slowly I got up and went downstairs. Josh, my eldest son, was sprawled in his ubiquitous sofa-lounging uniform – boxer shorts, T-shirt, and always just the one sock. He was watching TV and looked up as I came in.

'You all right, Mum?' he asked.

I nodded unconvincingly. But Josh wasn't fooled.

'Is it that doctor who's got it in for you?'

I hadn't told the children the details of the charges I was facing. I didn't want them to worry. But it's amazing what kids pick up.

'Yes, darling – but I'm okay.'

'Come here.' He reached out his arm and moved across, making room for me to lie next to him on the sofa.

I snuggled in against him and he smoothed back my hair as I rested my head on his arm. I was uncomfortable but I didn't want to move and disturb this rare moment of calm and closeness. After a few minutes, I noticed the pressure on my head was increasing with each stroke. I craned my eyes up to look at him and realised he was having to push my hair right down so he could continue watching *The Walking Dead* over the top of my head. I laughed and sat up. Somehow, my professional problems didn't seem to matter quite so much anymore.

I had my team and my family behind me. I felt strongly that I had the fact that I was 'right' behind me too. Now I had to hope that justice would be done.

CHAPTER 10

Trial

A nd so one rainy day in January, Nick knocked at my door.

'Time to go, Laura,' he said cheerfully.

He had kindly agreed to attend the trial with me as moral support. I was in need of it – although I would never have admitted this. Doctors tend not to ask for personal help. I think it is a deep cultural habit, picked up through years of brutal humiliation as students and being overworked on the wards. It makes you tough. You wear your emotional stunting like a badge of honour. 'I made it through. I've no feelings left. Now I'm just really fucked up.'

We got in the car and drove to a small town in West Sussex. It was raining and cold, but I realised I was sweating and my breathing was shallow. My body was alive with a fine tremor. I felt charged, as though I could take off my heeled shoes and run a hundred metres in eight seconds.

We checked into the Reception of a modern brick building. Inside, it had the terrible palette of most institutional headquarters: a sort of dull lime green and mustard yellow. The place was already starting to disintegrate: bits of Sellotape held lopsided messages written in marker pen on doors that didn't shut properly anymore.

We were told to sit on a couple of chairs at the bottom of some stairs. We were handed hastily written name badges on which my name was incorrectly spelled: Dr Laura Andrew Marshall. Not too impressive, but I found I didn't care. I could hardly speak. I was using all my concentration to sit calmly and hide the extremity of feeling in my body.

A woman with bouncy dark hair came down the stairs and tried to be friendly and reassuring.

'The panel is just going through the papers,' she said with forced cheer. I felt a wave of nausea come over me. I excused myself and went to the toilet. I spent a few minutes running my hands under cold water and breathing at my reflection in the mirror. I tried to relax my shoulders.

'Come on, Laura,' I said out loud to the terrified woman in the glass.

I stepped outside. The bouncy-haired lady said something and started walking up the stairs. Nick got up and squeezed my hand. I followed her. She led me along a darkly carpeted corridor and knocked on a closed door, which had a 'meeting in progress' sign on it.

'Come in,' said a male voice.

She opened the door and we walked in.

There were three men sitting on the other side of an oval table. They had their backs to the window. One of the men stood up and reached over the table to shake my hand and introduce himself. He was a GP. He then turned and introduced the other two. I nodded at them.

The man to his left was a pharmacist from another CCG's Medicine Management Team – their equivalent of Rachel. The man to his right was another GP. They were all in their late fifties, maybe even early sixties, I noticed. Straight away, that bothered me. While some GPs are wise and broad-minded, others are definitely 'old school'. If this panel belonged to the rigid protocol-driven camp, then I would be in for a rough ride.

The room was only just bigger than the table. I squeezed into my seat. There was palpable tension in the air. The central doctor tried to alleviate it by making a joke about the room. I couldn't follow and smiled weakly, struggling to control my racing mind.

Nick's voice said something from behind me. I hadn't realised he'd followed me inside. Then he sat down next to me. The dark-haired woman also sat down at one end of the table 'to transcribe the meeting'. I could feel cold sweat running down the inside of my shirt, tracking down my back almost to my waist. My dark jacket felt tight on my shoulders.

They started by asking some relatively straightforward questions.

'So, Laura, you work in Brighton,' began the doctor to the right. He looked down at the bunch of documents in front of him. 'At the… Brighton Health and Wellbeing Centre?'

'Yes, that's right.'

'And you have been a GP for a number of years?'

'Yes, for seventeen years.'

The pharmacist raised an eyebrow. I didn't know how to interpret his expression.

'Have you seen the allegations against you?' he asked.

'Yes, I have.'

Then we got into the meat of the 'meeting'. I presented my case. I could hear myself speaking cold, clinical sentences in a voice I barely recognised as my own. The men listened and nodded. They asked about our prescribing team and the strategies we had in place around addictive medication. They asked about Karen and my attitude and reasoning behind her Armour Thyroid prescription. They reeled off the long list of GMC allegations brought against me by the MMT.

Then there was silence. My mind was blank. I couldn't take it in. It all felt so unreal.

Now they were talking among themselves. I sat staring at the table. It had a smooth grey plastic surface. There were small white scratch marks on it. I wondered suddenly if they were made by the clawing fingernails of the doctors here before me.

But when I looked up, all three of them were smiling. I felt Nick's hand on my back.

'Laura, are you okay?' he asked me. I couldn't answer. I couldn't speak at all.

'Laura – they are dismissing the case. They don't think you have done anything wrong. They are going to talk to the MMT. It's over.'

I burst out crying, and once I started, I couldn't stop. Emotion poured out of me in a huge, overwhelming wave. Nick was trying to hug me. I could see two of the suited men over his shoulder. They clearly didn't know what to do and sat there frozen in embarrassment at my unusual display. I tried to pull myself together.

'Are you okay?' one of them asked kindly. I nodded between giant sobs. There was snot coming out of my nose.

'You should never have been put through this,' he told me.

We said our goodbyes. Unsurprisingly, no one wanted to shake my tear-soaked, snotty hand, but that was okay. Nick and I drove back to work.

Three weeks later, the PAG report came out. They had decided that the GMC's allegations were 'unfounded'. I could stay on the performers' list and was allowed to carry on prescribing Karen's Armour Thyroid, but Connor needed to change his fentanyl lollipops.

I called Connor to my surgery to tell him the bad news.

'I'm sorry, Connor. I tried.'

'I think it's gonna kill me,' he said bitterly.

'I'm sorry,' I repeated.

He nodded sadly. 'They don't believe me, do they?'

'They don't know you, Connor. It's not personal.'

He smiled up at me, a wry smile. 'Computer says no!' he observed.

'Yes, I'm afraid so. Computer says no.'

Slowly, relentlessly, ruthlessly, we brought his prescription down. Five lollipops a day for two weeks, then four, then three, and so on. He lied to us and told us he had lost his weekly prescription. Then he said he had to go away and needed more than one week's worth – but we saw him furtively shopping in the local Sainsbury's. His addiction and the emotional pain he was in were controlling him. We already knew that other painkillers wouldn't allow him to feel any benefits, but he agreed to take an antidepressant suggested by the pain team. It didn't work.

Six months later, Connor wasn't using fentanyl lollipops any longer. The MMT budget had been reduced. In the greater scheme of things, though, it wasn't reduced by very much. Whether it was related to stopping his fentanyl or not we will never really know, but Connor's relationship had deteriorated owing to his worsening moods and he had been forced to move out of his house and onto the streets. His swollen legs got repeated infections from sleeping sitting up and not washing. His kidneys had all but stopped working. His hospital stays had quadrupled due to his rapidly failing health, and if he survived his long stays in ITU, he was going to need council-funded housing.

Of course, the costs of all this far exceeded the cost of fentanyl lollipops. No money was saved by this course of action – in fact, money was wasted. Connor has had preventable suffering inflicted upon him. There's been no success – just a tragic inability to see the bigger picture and to help a vulnerable man in a way that actually works.

Fentanyl is a 'dirty drug' that should only be used in extreme cases – but those cases do exist. Applying unbending universal 'laws' cannot work in medicine. There are no absolutes here.

*

When I emerged from the PAG hearing, Nick dropped me straight back at the practice. I didn't want to take a break – in fact, it was a massive relief to lose myself in the normality of an afternoon at work.

'Ellen's coming in later, Laura,' said Rachel the moment I walked into Reception. 'Don't worry – Shilpa says we've got plenty of clonazepam!'

I burst out laughing. 'Oh bless her. I wonder what's the matter this time.'

'And Delilah was on the phone about her prescription.'

'Is she still okay?' I asked.

'Surprisingly enough – I think she is.'

I walked into my consulting room and sat in the quiet for a moment. The framed picture of my children smiled out at me from a long-distant holiday, oblivious then, as they are now, to the struggles and machinations of my life as a doctor. Gary heard I was back and flung open the door. He gave me a massive hug and a 'well done' before hurrying off to deal with a patient who was waiting to see him. I started up the computer and looked down my list for the afternoon. I was suddenly filled with pride at what we had created. For the first time in many weeks, I felt a deep sense of calm.

CHAPTER 11

Death and life

'To die will be an awfully big adventure.'

— J.M. BARRIE, PETER PAN

I was trying to obscure as much of the dead man's face as possible.

If I tipped my clipboard up at a certain angle, I could see the exposed sinews and the thin, grey cords of nerve and blood vessel, but not the eyes or the distorted mouth. I wished people died with a gentle smile on their faces, in peace, while their soul floated up to heavenly milk and honey. Instead, most of the dead heads I had seen wore contorted expressions of horror, mouths open and twisted as if paralysed in a desperate last shout. I always hated the heads. A hand or a foot was easier work, until you looked up casually, forgetting where you were, and saw the frozen face silently screaming at you.

We were medical students at our first dissection session. A young trainee surgeon talked us through the room and the set-up. These were our benches, these were our buckets for 'bits' and our tools: scalpels, forceps and, rather brilliantly, a 'groove director'. (The name makes me think of a DJ from the 1990s: let's hear it for the groove director, on the ones and twos, put your hands in the air, come on, let's go!)

Southampton University was a progressive university in those days. We did not have our own cadaver to work on, as traditional medical schools did. Instead, we worked on already partially dissected bodies. The surgeon explained that this was to 'save time'.

He walked us over to a big yellow bin. It looked like one of the large rubbish bins you find on the street nowadays that connect to the rubbish truck as it comes through. It had a heavy lid and on the side someone had stuck a horizontal A4 piece of paper, which had the word 'legs' written on it in coloured biro. The surgeon heaved the lid open – and the student next to me fainted. There is something deeply upsetting about dismembered parts of the human body, and a whole vat of them was traumatising for the uninitiated. I was careful to stand well back as we approached the 'head' container. As the lid was lifted, I mentally crossed 'head and neck surgeon' off my list of career options.

I spent the next few hours exposing and identifying the blood vessels of the foot. Then I set off home to the house I shared with three fellow students in the cheap end of town. As I was sitting on the bus on the way back, everyone I saw seemed to morph into a corpse before my eyes. An old man was sitting in the front seat, looking out of the window. As I studied him, his face seemed to drain of colour and develop that cold, grey hue of tissue in formaldehyde. His mouth dropped and twisted, his eyes rolled. I looked away quickly, glancing at the large man reading the paper next to me. The same thing happened. I was afraid to look at a mother and her two children sitting further back. I didn't want to see them with my metamorphosising death stare.

I found out later that what happened to me on the bus is not uncommon for medical students. When we encounter death, we don't always know how we'll respond.

I have since borne witness to many deaths. They have all been unique and important. Death, like birth, is charged with emotion and holds a mystery and an enormity that is completely humbling.

Mary, my patient who died from metastasising breast cancer, fought against her death right up to the end. Dylan Thomas's poem was very apt for her. He wrote of his father's death:

Do not go gentle into that good night,
Rage, rage against the dying of the light.

Many people die as they have lived, and Mary was one of them. She met her death with fire and energy and fight.

Frank, who asked me to release him, and Julie, who taught me so much at the beginning of my journey into Integrated Medicine, were very different. Both came to the end of their lives with calm. Their deaths were easier to watch, as a bystander; their last moments were almost beautiful. There was a sense of something unknown, unknowable, eternal.

But it's not always like that.

Najwa Khoury was tiny. At her tallest, she can't have been more than five foot. As she got older, her back rounded like a tree on a stormy shoreline, bent over by the constant force of the wind. She was no more than four foot ten inches by the time I met her. Her flat was in a row of terraced housing near to the sea by the main road that traversed the coast of Sompting, in one of the few buildings that was made up of more than one storey. These houses, already small enough as they were, had been further split up to create worryingly cramped living quarters.

I had been sent to see her by Harry, my GP trainer at the time. It would be good experience for me to 'see a death through', he had said. The house was covered in grey pebble dashing, in an attempt to reduce the need for maintenance. However, the fierce sea winds and salt spray had made short work of it. There were cracks showing down the front of the building and some pieces of windowsill were missing altogether. It didn't look like a particularly nice place to die.

I held my doctor's bag close to me as I rang the doorbell and stood back to see if there was any life within. The loose net curtain in the upstairs window twitched and then settled. Shortly afterwards, a tall, handsome man answered the door. He had short black hair and dark eyes.

'Hello, doctor, please come in.'

He had a distinctive Arabic accent. As he spoke, he nodded his head slightly in a respectful gesture. I followed him up the narrow stairs and into the top flat. It felt warm and calm in contrast to the busy road and windy air outside. We turned into the front room. There were small sofas arranged to form three sides of a square around a little fireplace, above which a richly coloured poster of the Virgin Mary had been carefully stuck to the wall. On either side there hung strings of wooden beads with little metal crosses at the bottom. To the right of the poster there was a shelf that was packed with neatly arranged My Little Ponies, their multicoloured manes smoothed and brushed. Each sofa was covered in a thick blanket with a garish, technicolour image on it. Sitting bolt upright on the middle sofa was an elderly lady with short hair and big dark-rimmed glasses. She looked like a little owl as she twisted her head around to greet us, her huge, magnified eyes blinking in welcome.

She started speaking quickly in Arabic in a tone that I recognised as being quite formidable. Another large young man, who had been sitting next to her as I walked in the room, hurriedly got up and moved towards me.

'Doctor, doctor, thank you so much for coming, please have a seat.'

The tirade of Arabic continued from his mother, fluctuating up and down and finally ending with a short staccato finish.

The man swallowed, glancing slightly nervously back at her.

'Would you like a cup of tea?' he stammered.

Before I could answer, the man who had let me in interjected.

'This is my brother, Bachir; my name is Fadi; we are Najwa's sons.'

I was about to reply when Najwa started off again. This time the torrent was directed at me.

'She wants you to sit down next to her,' offered Bachir helpfully.

I immediately sat down.

I was deeply impressed with how such a tiny person could emit such powerful authority. At a swift glance from their mother, Bachir and Fadi sat on the two remaining sofas. What ensued remains one of the most challenging experiences of translation I have ever encountered.

Every question I directed to Najwa would trigger a long, heated Arabic debate, which would then be distilled by one of the brothers, often to a yes/no answer.

The question 'Do you have any pain Najwa?' triggered about three minutes of discussion, throughout which Najwa was pointing at her sons and shouting loudly. In the end Fadi turned to me and replied: 'No.'

I managed to ascertain that Najwa had developed lung cancer in Palestine. Shortly after her diagnosis her husband was murdered, and her two sons had been forced to gather up their mother and flee to the UK. They had been here for approximately four months. They had seen the respiratory team and had been told that her cancer was not curable. Najwa had been offered some palliative chemotherapy to try to delay the rapid growth of the large tumour that occupied the lower third of her left lung. She knew it had spread to her spine and liver, but the family were not ready to accept that this was the end for Najwa. The sons were concerned that their mother had become considerably more breathless and was coughing up blood. This was a new thing, they explained. They wanted to start the chemo-therapy as soon as possible.

As I knelt on the floor to examine Najwa and take her blood, her sons stood over her, watching tentatively. Their eyes moved from her to me, trying to read something in my expression that might give away some important clue about their mother's health and prognosis. At this stage in my career I had not had much exposure to cancer that was this far progressed and really wasn't sure how much time was left, so it wasn't hard to keep a neutral expression.

As I left, both the sons followed me to the door.

'I will call you in a few days with the blood-test results and when I have spoken to the oncology team.'

'Thank you, doctor, thank you.'

As I drove back to the practice, I wondered who brushed the manes of the My Little Ponies.

Over the next few months I became a fairly frequent visitor to the Khoury family. Najwa had several rounds of chemotherapy but the tumour was aggressive and paid little attention to the chemical onslaught that was unleashed upon it. She weakened and took to her bed. The poster of the Virgin Mary and the rosary beads were moved into her bedroom and carefully pinned above her head.

I learnt that Bachir and Fadi had literally taken it in turns to carry their ailing mother across Lebanon, Turkey and then into Eastern Europe and up towards the UK. They were lucky they had made it here alive, but their asylum application was under consideration. For the moment they were allowed to work but it was an uncertain existence, stuck between two hostile worlds. Fadi had managed to get work at a mobile-phone shop; he had been an electrical engineer in Palestine. Bachir had recently been joined by his wife, Yara, and daughter, Camilla, who had made a similarly distressing journey.

'It was hard,' Bachir had told me. I wasn't sure what part exactly he was referring to but, in truth, it all sounded hard.

As Najwa grew weaker the Palliative Team and district nurses came to see her. A few days after their visit one of the nurses called me. She was clearly upset.

'Laura, you need to sign the Do Not Resuscitate form and leave it in the folder. I have discussed it with the family, but they won't agree to a DNAR order. You will have to do it. Najwa is going to die soon and it will be awful if the paramedics have to attempt CPR and take her to hospital. Poor lady, it will be so traumatic.'

'Why won't they sign it?'

'They say that their religion forbids it. They want to save her life – to have active treatment.'

'Okay, I'll go and see them.'

I had not encountered this situation before. Patients in hospital usually died during active treatment, or were sent home to die. This was an aspect of General Practice I had not been prepared for.

As I drove towards the house, I started planning the words that I would use in my head; I knew from experience they would be of the utmost importance in this sort of discussion. Conversations like this had backfired on me a few times before. As a medical student in my final year, I had been fixated on not forgetting to ask patients who were suffering with mental health disorders if they had suicidal thoughts. It was a notoriously difficult subject to broach, but one that was important in ascertaining their mental state. On one occasion I had sat attentively listening to one lady's description of her traumatic life before asking, 'Have you ever thought of killing yourself?' Unfortunately, it had sounded more like a suggestion than a question when it came out of my mouth. I hoped I would do better this time.

It was a warm May day and the sun was shining into the south-facing front room at Najwa's house. Camilla was sitting on the floor playing with her ponies and singing.

Bachir, Fadi and Yara had all met me at the door. They looked anxious and exhausted. They led me into Najwa's bedroom and stood back as I approached the small body under the covers.

Najwa had lost a lot of weight and looked more like a fallen, injured sparrow than the bright, powerful owl I had first encountered. Her breathing was heavy and laboured and each inhale was accompanied by a deep rasping noise. There was a light sheen on her skin and her eyes were closed. She had streaks of blood on her shirt.

I knelt down next to the bed and stroked her forearm, gently saying her name. She stirred slightly and opened her eyes and looked at me. There was a hint of recognition and a faint smile. She started to try to sit up, but the effort triggered a coughing fit, which wracked her whole body with brutal vibrations and brought with it droplets of bright red blood that spattered down her clothes. Bachir and Fadi moved quickly beside her and Yara picked up a clean shirt. Deftly they calmed her and changed her top.

I went through the motions of examining her and ascertained that she was really very close to the end. Her family stood behind me, watching this once-forceful figure fighting for breath.

Yara motioned to me to move into the front room so we could talk. We took our seats on the three sofas, Camilla's little singsong voice drifting up from behind them.

They all looked at me expectantly; I knew that what I said next would be important. I took a deep breath.

'Your mother is dying.'

There was a short pause before they all exploded into what looked like an intense argument that culminated with Bachir leaving the room shaking with anger, tears rolling down his face. Yara followed him.

Fadi and I were left sitting on the sofas. It was hot, and I was starting to feel beads of sweat on the back of my neck. Fadi sat looking at the floor for a few moments before he left the room too. I was about to get up and leave the flat. I had clearly completely blown our best chance of helping this loving and brave family come to terms with their mother's situation. They had carried her so far in the hope of saving her – of course it would be impossible for them to accept her death.

Just as I was about to stand up, they came back in and sat down. They looked calm as Bachir spoke.

'What is the best thing we can do for her now?'

Steadying my voice, I took a moment to think about my reply.

'I think the best thing we can do is to make her death as comfortable and peaceful and happy as possible.'

I waited, hoping against hope this would land okay. They talked briefly, nodding, and then turned to me.

'Is it better that we are with her or should she be left alone to be in peace?' Fadi asked.

Again, I thought for a moment.

'When she was sick before, did she like to be alone and quiet or did she like to be in the middle of things?'

They seemed to relate to this. Fadi and Bachir were smiling as they chatted for a few minutes before Fadi turned back to me.

'She always wanted to be in the middle of things, bossing us all around.'

'Yes, I can believe that.' I smiled

'What will happen now?' said Bachir

'I think she will probably get weaker and her breathing will get harder. We can give her medicine in a pump, which will help to keep her calm and comfortable. If you are worried about anything, call me or the nurses. The numbers are in the folder. You don't need to call the ambulance at all.'

We sat for a minute.

'We have another brother; he was lost in the fighting, but we think he will be here soon. He's tried to contact us. We think he is in France.' Fadi said.

'Does Najwa know that?' I asked.

'Yes, we think so.'

'Maybe she is waiting for him – that happens sometimes.'

They nodded.

After I had left, I spoke to the Palliative Care Team.

'Did you leave the DNAR form in the folder?' they asked. I dodged the question and we moved on to discussing medication.

I will do it later, I thought. At least I had given them a plan of what to do if she died; a plan that did not involve the paramedics.

Several days later I received a call from Fadi. Their brother had arrived the day after I had seen them, and Najwa had died within a few hours. They had all been around her, talking to her.

After she'd died, they had called the nurses who had come and helped them with the body and with what to do next.

I was grateful I had never had to sign a form that they did not want signed.

*

Grant approached his death as he approached his life – with absolute control. He'd had to keep a careful grip on his affairs as a young man. In the 1970s, he had been a radical gay activist and journalist, and this had brought him into contact with the law. His flat in Bloomsbury had been raided many times and he was no stranger to the inside of a police cell. As society moved forwards and changed its perspective, he'd moved from criminal to hero. He had to watch his back for different reasons then.

He'd had many partners, but all of them had left him. There were different reasons given, but I guessed that underlying all the stories, the same cause kept repeating: Grant's unbending will. What Grant wanted, Grant got. He didn't easily accommodate others. Perhaps the persecutions of his early life had stayed with him, preventing him from ever backing down.

As he grew older, he became extremely overweight. With that came the ills of diabetes, heart disease and arthritis. His mobility reduced to a few steps, but his will and ingenuity kept him engaged and active. He commandeered an office chair with wheels to enable him to scoot around his kitchen preparing large and indulgent meals. Living in a ground-floor flat meant that he could roll his chair to the front door, then in a few heavy and painful steps, he would lurch outside to his car.

To the uninformed eye, his flat looked like the most appalling tip. To him, however, it represented the rich history of his life. Papers and old magazines teetered in piles against every wall. Ornaments, awards and trophies covered the surfaces. A thick layer of grease lay over the kitchen. Small patches of the bathroom were clean – but the rest did not bear close scrutiny.

There were disagreements over his care. The district nurses wanted him to go into a nursing home, but he refused. That would have been the ultimate humiliation for him. They tried to get a hospital bed for him but he refused that too, hanging grimly on at home.

He called me to visit him one day. He was sitting in his large TV chair and had clearly been doing so for some considerable time. It was as if he and the chair had become one unified being. His swollen legs were cracked and fluid from them was leaking onto the floor. His abdomen spilled out from under his shirt and merged into the soft brown leather. He was sweating profusely and breathing hard. His skin was puffy and sallow and his forehead was clenched in a deep frown. He was the epitome of misery.

As gently as I could, I checked his vital signs. His heart was now unable to cope with the job of pushing his blood around his body. Plasma from the barely moving blood in his lungs was seeping out of the vessels and into the lung spaces. He was drowning. I pulled the office chair up next to him and sat by his side.

'Hi, Grant.'

'Hi.' He barely managed to get the word out between breaths.

'Grant, you don't look very comfortable. Can we help you? Can we get you into a better position? We could put a hospital bed in the bedroom? I think you would feel better.'

He shook his head vehemently.

'It's over. I'm dying. I don't want to... go through this.' He paused to catch his breath. 'Can't you – can't you help me? I just want to go now. Can't you do... that?'

I felt the tears spike at the back of my eyes. His suffering was intense, palpable. One of my early GP trainers once told me how the nursing homes would call him in the night when people were like this, 'To put them out of their misery.' He would give them morphine and they would die, peacefully and quickly. Not anymore. The infamous case of Harold Shipman, a GP who was arrested in 1998 for murdering hundreds of his elderly patients, put paid to that. After Dr Shipman's abuse of his position was exposed, far closer checks were introduced on medication decisions.

But Grant was right. It was game over. The twenty-six medications he was taking could no longer help him. Nothing could. His kidneys and heart could not cope anymore and he had lost the will to drive them any further.

'I'm so sorry, Grant. I can't do that.'

He would have to suffer for a while longer.

We put up a syringe driver, a mechanised pump to deliver a constant supply of pain relief, to try to ease his grim last few days. He died sitting there, seeping into his chair. I still feel I let him down. I couldn't help him in the way that he wanted. The decision wasn't one that I could take.

*

In the early years of my career, I was terrified of death, error and the coroner's court.

Then slowly, as I was forced to face them all, they lost their foreboding. They became just part of things.

I learned that death is not the worst thing that can happen to us and was able to view it as another process of life. Sometimes it was an incredible relief, sometimes it was cruel and unjust. But sometimes it could be beautiful and profound. Whatever form a person's death took, it was made better if those involved engaged with it openly and wisely. Our tendency as a society is to shy away from the concept and process of death. But we do ourselves, our patients and our loved ones a great disservice in this.

Sometimes death is very quick – a sudden heart attack out of the blue or an accident – but often it takes time. There is some evidence to suggest that at the point of death there is a surge in endorphins and other chemicals, which can make dying an intensely euphoric and profound experience. Not everyone seems to go through this. But in my experience, people have more chance of finding an ecstatic moment at death if they have managed to positively engage with it. The process of dying can bring great peace and acceptance, if we let it.

A Swedish diplomat called Dag Hammarskjöld said: 'Do not seek death. Death will find you. But seek the road which makes death a fulfilment.'

*

Often it's in facing death that people find their true sense of meaning and purpose. But sometimes we are lucky enough to be shown this in life. I had this good fortune one evening in the unlikely surroundings of a gym changing room.

In my previous practice, there was a gym several blocks down from us. It was a small, independently owned establishment. They had several treadmills for running, along with cross trainers and step machines. In the corner was the scary free-weights area full of enormous men whose muscular arms were no longer able to rest fully flush to their bodies but stuck out at a slight angle. They had a studio for classes and two small, single-sex changing rooms with benches around the edges and clothes pegs in the walls to hang coats. It was a bit like an old-fashioned school changing room. There were no cubicles, nor any place for shyness.

A number of the staff who worked there were patients of ours. One of these was a young Polish woman called Eliza who was a fairly regular attendee at the practice owing to her high levels of anxiety around her health.

It was late in the evening. I'd done my thirty minutes on the cross trainer and had a shower. I was standing with my hair bundled up in a towel, rubbing moisturiser into the dry skin on my ankles. The changing room was empty, so I was not too bothered about my nakedness.

At that moment, Eliza came in.

'Ah, doctor!' she said. 'I thought I saw you come in.'

'Hi,' I replied.

'So, I've had this pain in my tummy for about three days now,' she immediately began. 'It's quite bad. I don't know what it is.'

I couldn't help myself. Automatically, I started the history-taking process.

'Oh – okay. Have you had any other symptoms?'

I kept on going down the list. I was like an automated machine.

'Any nausea or diarrhoea?'

After a few minutes, I stealthily reached out my hand and grabbed my pants from the top of my bag. Trying not to break the flow of the consultation, I managed to get my underwear on. This achieved, and feeling emboldened, I struggled into the rest of my clothes.

By the end of the consultation, I was fully dressed. I had also ascertained that Eliza was most likely suffering with the tail-end of mild gastroenteritis.

'Thank you, doctor,' she finished cheerily and left the changing room. I gathered up my stuff and hurried out before anyone else arrived for a quick check-up.

That was when I realised the truth about myself. When every single thing has been removed from me – even my clothes – I am still a doctor. The practice of medicine gets meshed into your core. It can be a painful process – but it's worth it.

Being a doctor is the essence of who I am, and it's who I always will be.

PART 4

Pandemic

CHAPTER 12

Warnings

Life goes on. It changes. There's no happy ending – just the next chapter starting.

Sometimes change happens gradually: the surface of the water stays smooth. But every now and then, a big wave hits. The one that upends everything, that throws the whole world into chaos.

Nothing exposes a fractured health and social care system, or tests a team of professionals to the limit, quite like a pandemic.

It's January 2020. I am on my way home. It's been a long and busy day. There is a storm coming. We know it. We can feel it. We are starting to prepare, to clear the decks, to change how we work.

It's still hard to see the storm clouds, but the wind has changed. It's coming from the east, via a ski chalet and a conference in Singapore. Covid arrives in Brighton in early February, just before half-term. Suddenly we hear on the news that a returning traveller carrying the virus is a local man. He has landed at Gatwick airport, then journeyed home by train. No doubt he hugged his friends and sent his kids off to school. He could have spread it widely.

COVID-19.

*

The year 2020 had such a good ring about it. It was going to be a great one – a new decade beginning, a fresh start. We made plans and resolutions. We woke up with hangovers and ridiculously good intentions. Then slowly, like an IV drip of futuristic imagery, came the first wave of information contagion. Coronavirus – born from the Wuhan wet markets, a virus from pangolins or long-eared bats or both. Some fearful new viral hybrid made on the stone market floors in the mixing blood of the world's most rare and endangered animals. Could this be nature's weapon – a protest against human encroachment on the natural world? Could it be nature's warning?

We receive directions from Public Health England and the local Clinical Commissioning Group to monitor all people coming back first from China, then from Singapore and Japan. Bulletins and guidance come thick and fast, and we discuss them at our daily morning meetings.

'It's definitely here,' Lolita Simcock points out. 'It's in the local community. We just can't see it yet.'

We all agree that this must be the case.

'But until there's some kind of national announcement, it's going to be difficult to get people to understand the risk,' she goes on worriedly.

'And there needs to be testing,' says Francis. 'Proper contact tracing, to try to contain it.'

But it's just not happening fast enough. Eventually, and probably too late, some contacts begin to be tracked down and isolated. GP practices are shut and disinfected. But no one is tested. Nothing else happens.

Next some fellow doctors and friends are put into quarantine for two weeks. Two weeks! It feels like an age. But where's the virus now? Where has it gone? All through February we wait, watching out for travellers from Asia but all the while knowing it is already here. It must be.

Then Italy falls. Next is Iran. And then Spain, and then France. In the UK, new cases start to arise with no clear traceable contact.

It's here for sure now. We start to see more respiratory symptoms in young people, but still we are only supposed to be watching out for patients with a positive contact or recent travel to affected areas. Like a tanker that takes weeks to respond, the government's guidelines lag behind the reality on the ground.

Frantic messages appear on medical forums and Facebook groups from colleagues in Europe, warning us to act. We start to talk about creating a 'dirty' room in the practice and having 'dirty staff'. Patients suspected of carrying the virus will be treated there, and only there. Those who treat them will follow strict containment protocols. We think seriously about PPE – Personal Protective Equipment. We order twenty pairs of goggles from Amazon and some hazmat suits from eBay. I feel like there is a good chance I am completely overreacting, but they are only £8 so we order four. Pretty soon I wish we'd ordered more.

On 9 March, a patient is booked into my surgery. He phoned the NHS 111 advice line and was told to see a GP within four hours. He is young and tall. His dark hair is slightly matted at his neck and he is sweating. He looks ill. He starts to tell me his history but breaks into a spasm of dry coughing that he struggles to stop. His temperature is high at 38°C, but his oxygen saturations are 99 per cent and he is talking without having to breathe more quickly. I check his respiratory rate: sixteen breaths per minute, pulse ninety-eight. His chest sounds clear.

I decide he does not need hospital admission, but I am pretty sure he is a possible COVID-19 patient. I ask him to go home and isolate for seven days and say that his housemate must do so for fourteen days. I tell him I will organise a Covid test and let him know how it will be done. He apologises for coming in, but it's not his fault.

We disinfect the room and I wash my hands and wonder what to do with my clothes, which are probably saturated with the virus. Eventually I change into my gym clothes, which are in my bag, and put my other clothes in a hazard bag. I think I will have to boil them later. On second thoughts, I doubt that my prized new shirt will survive being boiled, so I opt to leave everything in the bag for seventy-two hours, until the virus dies.

I find the latest guidelines from Public Health England on the government website. It directs me to the local Health Protection Service. They in turn direct me to a lab in Southampton, but when I call them, they won't speak to a GP. I phone the local hospital lab, and they don't know what to do either. So I call PHE and eventually speak to someone who asks if the patient has either been in direct contact with a COVID-19 patient, or recently travelled to the areas where the disease has been identified. 'No,' I reply, 'but his history and symptoms were pretty convincing.'

They won't test him. It's not in their guidelines.

I call the patient; he is angry and really concerned. I give him some antibiotics, just in case I am missing a bacterial infection, and promise to call him every day to check his breathing. If he gets worse, he is to call me back or call 999. He follows an unusual course of illness – one that will start to feel familiar to us clinicians over the next few months.

This is a strange virus, with a long tail of lasting symptoms. The patient is more unwell than he appears. His symptoms fluctuate over the next ten days, better then worse, his temperature going up and down, rising in the afternoon and evening. He gets very out of breath on walking for a few weeks after his main symptoms go. But he has no test at any time and neither do any of his contacts, including me.

We have a practice meeting on the morning after I have seen him.

'Right,' I say, 'it's here, and it's moving quickly. From now on, we're going to act as though it's widespread in the community. First of all, that means that vulnerable staff should go home. Jacqui, please can you put together a system for disinfecting the "dirty" room? Maureen, can Reception start cancelling non-urgent appointments, please?'

Maureen looks unhappy. I understand why: we certainly don't like to do this. But we know that we must. The sense of emergency is building. Around me, my team swings into action. Jacqui gets to work on strict cleaning policies. I can hear the Reception staff hitting the phones. We start to carry out as many consultations as we can by telephone. Our therapists follow suit. As far as possible, we move groups online: singing, creative arts, meditation. Of course, it's not the same: taking part now depends on people's access to the internet, and also on their comfort with technology. Some patients take to it like ducks to water, while others struggle.

It is confusing for everyone, and for a week or so we struggle to change our entrenched habits. We discover a great phone app on our computer system that lets us consult on a video link. The only downside is that your own image appears on the screen too. I find this very off-putting, and frankly demoralising. It's hard not to look at the wrinkles you have developed, or the grey strands in your hair. I prefer the image of myself that exists vaguely in my head. She is at least fifteen years younger and very much better all-round than the unfamiliar talking head that sits below my patients on the screen.

The official PPE order arrives. Now at least we have some surgical masks and aprons and gloves. Public Health England issues new PPE guidance suggesting that surgical masks are in fact fine to use with infected patients unless you are doing 'an aerosol-generating procedure'. They mean procedures like flushing someone's lungs on the Intensive Care Unit. But surely someone coughing is aerosol-generating? We are not convinced by their guidance.

On the news, we keep seeing images of well-covered healthcare workers in Wuhan. Our flimsy masks and aprons don't look like they are going to cut it. I try the masks on: my breath flows seamlessly out around the edges and with it, potentially, millions of viral particles. It does not feel safe. All our usual suppliers are completely out of PPE. NHS England bought the lot, they tell us. Our usual sources can't get hold of any. No gowns, no FFP3 masks (the safer variety), no visors or scrubs.

'Right – we must take action on this,' says Gary briskly. 'We'll source the supplies we need ourselves, not keep waiting for them to be provided.'

I agree, and we decide to try social media. I ask a friend to send out a Twitter request for equipment and like manna from heaven, bits and pieces filter in. A closed dentist surgery donates the FFP3 masks, local mothers bring in their children's full-face snorkelling masks and another friend uses her 3D-printer to produce the filters to attach. A neighbour uses the same method to make visors. We're still worried, but buoyed up by the support that we're receiving. The hazmat suits arrive from eBay.

It gets busier and busier in the practice. There are only three doctors and two nurses left who are able to see patients. Alongside a handful of Reception and admin staff, we make a tiny crew. We have 15,500 patients on our list, some of whom are in nursing homes or housebound and very vulnerable, reliant on carers and relatives. People are starting to panic, stockpiling medicine and loo roll (why loo roll?) Shilpa is inundated with requests for asthma inhalers and months' worth of medications. There is a strong vein of anxiety in most consultations. People are worried about themselves, worried about losing their jobs, their homes, their loved ones.

It feels like the first wave of this catastrophe is a contagious fear that is surging through communities. We spend twelve- to thirteen-hour days on the phone and visiting patients at home, getting good at 'donning' and 'doffing' our PPE in the windy streets and people's porches. But our main focus is on our nursing-home patients. These are the most vulnerable people – these are the sitting ducks. Sam sets up a rota to attend our main nursing home daily.

Two days later, he calls me on his mobile. He has just finished a visit. A patient there has developed a high fever and cough.

'They don't have PPE,' he says to me. 'We left our one pair of scrubs with them and it was stolen immediately. The staff are terrified.'

'Can we give them some equipment?' I reply.

'We can try.' He sounds flat and low. 'It's more than that, though. Staff are being told not to wear it unless the patient has tested positive.'

'But that's crazy,' I say. 'They're not testing anyone in the community so... ' I pause '... that means they won't use PPE with anyone.'

'I know,' he replies. There is a silence on the phone. 'They are all going to die, Laura.' His voice breaks.

'Let's just take the nursing homes all the PPE we can and ask the nurses to wear it on the sly with all patients. We have to try to do the right thing.'

'Agreed,' he says.

The next day Derek, the unwell patient at the nursing home, gets a golden test. It's positive. He has been in the home for over three weeks. That means he must have caught coronavirus from someone in there.

I call Sam. 'Are they wearing PPE?'

'Only with Derek,' he replies. 'They are worried they will run out. And the nurses are worried they'll be sacked if they go against the guidelines they've been given, which is not to wear... ' He trails off.

'We *know* he caught it on the ward. That means they *must* use PPE with everyone. They must assume it's come from one of the staff, or other patients,' I reply.

'They won't do it. They are scared.' He sounds exhausted. He had to FaceTime Derek's family on his phone. He described holding his mobile up close to Derek so he could speak to his wife and daughter. Derek never saw them face to face again. He died five days later. Alone.

'You better go home,' I say. 'I'm so sorry, Sam. I will try to call the CCG and see if they can help the nurses understand they won't lose their jobs if they wear the PPE we gave them.'

The next morning, I manage to speak to the chair of the CCG.

'I'm sorry, Laura, my hands are tied. Guidelines are guidelines,' he says to me.

'But the guidelines are wrong – you know that.' My frustration is boiling over.

'I'm sorry. There is nothing I can do,' he repeats. 'I will speak to our infection control nurse. Sorry.'

A few hours later we get an email from the infection control nurse reiterating the same inappropriate guidelines. It's desperately angering and frustrating.

*

I remember the remarkable story of what happened during Hurricane Katrina, the catastrophe that swept through Florida on 29 August 2005. When Katrina hit the coast, thousands of people were displaced from their homes overnight with nothing. The government agencies took weeks to mobilise their response. Process had to be followed, decisions signed off and guidelines drawn up and amended. And while strict protocol was blindly adhered to, people were starving and freezing, stranded on the roofs of their houses or in makeshift shelters. One thousand and eight-hundred and thirty-three people died.

At this extraordinary time, many lives were saved by the directors of the Walmart supermarket chain. The words of one of them come into my mind. 'Do the right thing and we will back you up.'

Walmart gathered its staff together and told them:

'A lot of you are going to have to make decisions above your level. Make the best decision that you can with the information that's available to you at the time, and above all, do the right thing.'

With this agency and autonomy, the Walmart staff went out into the local stores and gave out food and sanitary products in exchange for handwritten notes of payment, or just on trust. They had delivered millions of dollars of aid before the government tanks and provisions even left their stations.

The author and WHO advisor Atul Gawande reviewed the Walmart action and concluded:

'In other words, to handle this complex situation, they did not issue instructions. Conditions were too unpredictable and constantly changing. They worked on making sure that people talked. Given common goals to do what they could to help and coordinate with one another, Walmart's employees were able to fashion some extraordinary solutions.'

Like the new vessels that grow around blocked arteries in the heart, lifelines of supply will develop to keep the heart muscle of society working. They just need to be enabled, and not restricted.

*

Over the next few days, we take scrubs made out of duvet covers, and 3D-printed visors and masks and sanitiser, into the nursing home. The nurses start to wear their PPE at all times. But the virus has already spread. Three patients have died and many of the staff have gone off sick. There's still a severe lack of testing, so the true extent of the disease there may never be known.

On my way home one evening, I meet Dawn, the mother of a little boy my daughter went to nursery with. She looks worn out. She is still wearing the blue uniform of her carers' company. I know that she is part of a team of dedicated care workers who care for frail and vulnerable people in their own homes. She is one of those people who seems to be deeply good. My mother would say, 'If you cut her in half, she would be good through and through.' She is walking slowly and deliberately, looking at her phone. I call out to her and we stop a good two metres apart and exchange 'hellos'.

She asks me about my work and congratulates me on the great job I am doing. I witter on about it being hard and exhausting, about the lack of PPE and testing. I tell her about my Twitter campaign and my cobbled-together ensemble of visor and hazmat suit. She laughs and says kindly how clever she thinks I am to have been able to do that.

As we are parting, I ask her about how she is getting on. She tells me she is one of two remaining carers out of the eleven who usually look after fifty patients in their homes. Twelve of her patients are suspected Covid-positive, and one of them has died. Her other nine colleagues are either self-isolating or unwell. One is hospitalised with the disease.

She has no PPE at all. She has visited six people today and washed them and fed them and changed them.

All across the country, fierce fights are being waged in Intensive Care Units and hospital wards. But the main, long battle lines of this viral war extend through the nursing homes, care homes, warden-controlled flats and sheltered accommodations that hold the old and vulnerable – out of sight and out of mind.

I feel humbled as I watch her walk away, the real hero of this new corona world.

CHAPTER 13

Strength

By late spring 2020, the warnings our European medical colleagues and others raised about the advancing coronavirus turn out to be more than justified. The new virus, officially known as SARS-CoV-2, or COVID-19, has spread rapidly across the country and across the world.

London and areas in the North of England are hit the worst. We tune in for bulletins every evening as the grim death toll rises. ITU consultants in scrubs and gowns stand outside their units talking of deaths – terrifying deaths in isolation. There are agonising stories from front-line workers of relaying messages to the sick from their loved ones. Initially relatives are denied entry to the COVID RED ZONES inside hospitals. These Red Zones are wards of Covid-positive patients with access restricted only to designated staff. No one else is allowed in. It will take many months for this rule to be changed and for families to be with their dying relatives.

The statistics for deaths that appear on our TV screens are huge. As humans, we evolved to live in small communities, and one effect of this is that we don't find it easy to make sense of huge numbers of people. As a result, the Covid reports can make it feel as if half the population is dying.

It is very hard to get information about the situation around us in Brighton. There are no published statistics for months and months.

Luckily for us, one of our newest practice nurses, Tara, is seconded into the county hospital. Tara is highly intelligent but recently qualified. Other than as a student, she has never worked on a hospital ward. When she gets the dreaded call announcing her transfer, she understandably feels terrified, but she attacks her new role with the resolve and determination of a true professional. Immediately, she applies herself to learning protocols she thought she would never need to know: how to manage dangerous intravenous drugs and infusions and advanced life-support training.

Soon she is working flat-out on an elderly care ward, which is supposed to be a GREEN ZONE – Covid-free – but then staff start going off with suspicious symptoms. Still no testing is available. Stress levels on the ward are high and people snap at each other. Tara tells me about what's happening, and I realise that I must try to help her. The two of us take more than one tearful, socially distanced walk together, during which I give her all the support and encouragement I can. This is a time to be brave.

But I know her experiences are traumatic. Like all medical professionals in the international emergency of COVID-19, she's stepping up, giving all she has to her work. But she is still a person, still vulnerable, still affected by what she's going through. She needs to process all of this – the horror and fear she is witnessing, her feeling of being pushed to the limit, of not being able to do enough to help. Unprocessed trauma can affect a person deeply, no matter how dedicated they are, or how tough.

*

There was one night in my paediatric training that I will never forget. In those days we had no debriefings or chances to reflect on events. Things just happened – and then you moved on. If it was a bad memory, you tried to forget about it, banish it from your brain. If it was good, you could keep it and come back to it when times were hard. No one offered you a chance to talk it through, to come to terms with it, to have a natural, human response.

That night, I was on call on the neonatal unit with a more senior registrar, Helen.

She was diligent, accomplished and hard-working. I liked being on call with her. She wouldn't shirk her work. She would come if you called her. It was nearly midnight and both of us were tired – we had started work at eight that morning. I could feel the tiny movement inside my own pregnant abdomen: little flutters that might easily be confused with movements of the intestine, except the quality of them was different, lighter, like the gentle brush of a finger on the back of your hand that can be felt deep inside you.

My bleep went off: the delivery suite. I walked to the nurses' desk where the phone was and dialled the number on my bleep. One of the midwives answered.

'We need you in room twelve. Looks like a stillbirth. Twenty-two weeks plus four days. No trace and she's well progressed in prem labour.'

'Okay,' I replied. 'Someone will be there in a minute.'

I walked back and spoke to Helen. We agreed that I would go to the delivery. It was almost certainly a formality having the paediatrician there: resuscitation of a baby less than twenty-four weeks old will almost certainly fail. It's also massively traumatic, and were it to be successful, there's near certainty of inflicting terrible damage. This baby was below the age that we would try to save its life. A situation like this was always worse if the foetus came out wriggling and alive. It was hard to watch it gasp for breath and struggle as it tried to drive its under-developed body to function in this alien environment. But in this case, we knew already that no trace of a heartbeat was present. This baby was not going to live.

I walked along the darkened corridor and took the stairs down to the labour ward. I found room twelve. The mother was on the bed. Her dark hair was matted over her face and she was craning her neck forward, lost in the throes of labour. Her husband stood next to her at the head of the bed, bending forward and trying to encourage her to push. Despite the drama of birth, there is usually a light atmosphere in the delivery room. The midwives often try to crack jokes and offer encouragement. There is back rubbing and faded smiles between the contractions. Everyone is focused on the coming new life.

Not in this room, though. Here, there was only fear. This was not the pain before the joy – this was just pain on pain. In between contractions, the woman turned and buried her face in her husband's chest, sobbing. Tears were running down his face too. My hand went instinctively to my own pregnant belly as I fired up the Resuscitaire. I laid a clean sheet out on the warmed mattress at the base and turned on the overhead heater. I went through the motions of checking the oxygen supply, the intubation tray, the suction tube. If the baby came out and cried, I would lay it on the mattress and wrap it up in the towel and sheet. I would check the pulse and respiratory effort. Then I would, most likely, give the baby to the mother and father to hold. They would have a very short time together as a family.

I turned back to the bed. The mother was screaming loudly now and hunched forward as she tried to push down. Her legs had been put up into stirrups and I could just see the foetal head starting to crown. Then suddenly, blood started oozing all around the head. I had witnessed the end of many deliveries, but this did not look right. The blood was starting to run more quickly now. I looked across at the obstetric registrar who had entered the room earlier and was now sitting on a stool between the woman's legs. I recognised him from the canteen that evening. He was tall and good-looking, with dark blond hair in a thick side parting. He was wearing pale green scrubs and he had short, white wellington boots on and gloves. He had looked so relaxed in the canteen, leaning back on his chair, chatting to his team and laughing. Now his face was taut with concentration.

The blood was running more freely and the mother was clearly in considerable pain. Every muscle in her body was tensed and contracted; she was making a loud, guttural sound. This was worlds away from the aromatherapy and candle-lit birth planning of antenatal classes. This was pure animal distress. Noise and pain and energy filled the room, thickening the air with emotion, making it hard to breathe.

The obstetrician was sweating and half-standing as blood poured onto the floor, splattering his boots and scrubs. His equipment trolley stood next to him, lined with the brutal devices of emergency delivery. He needed to get the baby out. His right hand was in the mother's vagina, trying to pull the lifeless head down towards him. He grabbed the large scissors, cut an episiotomy to widen the birth canal and then took the forceps and secured them around the baby's head. He pulled down, using all his might. Suddenly his arm shot back and he staggered, just managing to regain his balance as the bleeding escalated. The baby had been born, its body bloodied and crushed. He or she was dead. I didn't want to look. But the critical risk now was to the mother's life, from haemorrhage. The obstetrician's face was panicked. His eyes widened and he was breathing hard as the adrenalin coursed around his body.

'Prepare theatre!' he shouted.

There was a frenzy of activity. Midwives were flying around the room, propping open doors and kicking the brakes off the wheels at the base of the bed. The bed was mobilised, pushed down the corridor at a run, surrounded by noise and urgency. Then they were gone. I was left standing alone in the bloody room.

I stood there for a while, unable to move. The equipment trolley had been pushed back against the wall. I turned away from it, not wanting to see what lay in the grip of the forceps there: I had heard of pre-term babies being decapitated in the desperate effort to deliver them. I did not want that image in my mind. I stared down at the white sheet and towels lying over the warmed mattress. There were two tiny flecks of blood on it.

I knew that the room would soon be cleared, the tiny body removed, wrapped carefully and prepared in case the parents wanted to see it. Most mothers do, even in such harrowing circumstances: what we imagine is often worse than reality, and seeing the body of a loved one can be a way towards acceptance and peace. And to its mother, every baby is beautiful.

I powered off the Resuscitaire and waited until it was cold and shut down. I felt as though a little part of my soul had died and shut down with it. Looking straight ahead, I walked outside. I made my way unseeingly back along the corridor and up to my on-call room on the neonatal unit. The room was dark and the main light was broken. I had meant to tell the janitor about it earlier that day but had forgotten. Right now, it felt as though some other, completely different person could have cared about that.

I sat on the side of the bed staring down at my legs. I could just make out the blue of my scrubs in the half-light filtering in from the tall orange street lamps in the car park outside. After a few moments, I let my body fall to the left and pulled my legs up onto the little single bed. I must have drifted into an uneasy sleep.

The next thing I heard was the insistent noise of my bleep. I unclipped it from my waist and checked the number. Theatre one. I fumbled for the telephone on the side table by the bed and dialled the number.

'Morning!' came a cheery voice. 'We've got a crash section in theatre one. Failure to progress, no meconium, thirty-eight weeks. Trace has been good.'

'Okay,' I said. 'Okay. I'll be there in a sec.' This baby would be born at full term, healthy and strong.

I looked at the small square alarm clock on the side table: 4.45 a.m. Suddenly, from nowhere, a strong metallic taste filled my mouth. I just made it to the little basin in the corner of the room to throw up. I had been fortunate to have avoided morning sickness so far in my pregnancy; luckily this was only a thin, yellowish bile, which flushed easily down the plug hole. I caught my reflection in the cracked mirror above the basin. In the early-morning light, I looked a ghostly yellow colour. I looked away and splashed cold water on my face and then drank deeply from the tap. I could almost feel the cool liquid soaking into my cells, renewing and regenerating. I quickly brushed my teeth and walked down the corridor towards the theatre.

There was a large window at the end of the corridor, which looked out over Kingston Gate. Beyond it the green trees and grasslands of Richmond Park stretched out. The sun was just coming up, its early fingers of light pushing back the horrors of the night.

As I got down onto the labour ward, I could smell toast. Walking into theatre, I saw the obstetric registrar from last night 'scrubbing up', washing his hands with the dark brown betadine wash. He looked grey with exhaustion and his shoulders were stooped under the bright theatre lights. Another man in his early thirties was already at the operating table, forearms elevated to keep them clean and away from potential infection risk. I guessed he was a junior, learning his trade. A woman lay on the table, her large pregnant abdomen rising like a smooth mountain up from her legs and falling abruptly to her lower ribs. Her head was obscured by the green canvas screen used to prevent the mother and father from seeing the major operation going on in her unfeeling pelvis.

I took up my station at the Resuscitaire. It had already been turned on and the sheet and towels laid out on the warmed mattress. One of the midwives smiled at me kindly as I went through my habitual checks. This was business as usual. The obstetrician was chatting to the father and someone put a tinny radio on. It was the breakfast show; whoever was plucked out of this abdomen was going to be born to the dulcet tones of Chris Tarrant. I wondered if the infant might have lasting psychological damage.

This procedure was routine. A woman whose labour hadn't gone to plan would be quickly and safely helped to deliver. After a few minutes, a reassuringly large baby was lifted up and passed over to me. She was still a dusky colour and covered in white vernix. I laid her down on the little mattress under the overhead heater and gave her a brisk rub with the towels. Immediately her chest rose and she drew her first deep, powerful breath. Pink blood flooded through her body – and with that, I felt that little piece of cold, dead soul inside me warm back up to life. What I had witnessed that night began to lose its grip. I rubbed this beautiful newborn baby girl a little more. Once she was crying well, I wrapped her in the towels and sheet and turned to hand her to Mum.

Now I look across at Tara, her pale, taut expression, the tears that are starting in her eyes. She's just finished a shift among the victims of the pandemic. First thing in the morning, she'll be back to work another. I want to give her a hug, but we have to remain at a distance. All I have are words. I know that if she can express how it has been, get the feelings out of her instead of holding them inside, the horror and helplessness can start to leave her. No one ever spoke to me about what I saw in that delivery room. I was left, as we all were in those times, to deal with it entirely alone. I won't let this happen to Tara.

'Just tell me all about it,' I say to her. 'Take as much time as you need. I'm here to listen.'

*

Having Tara on duty at the Royal Sussex Hospital turns out to be helpful for another reason too. She can send us text messages with weekly updates, like smoke signals from allied troops.

'Seventy-one Covid inpatients, fourteen in critical care.'

'Fifty-five Covid inpatients, eleven in critical care.'

At the practice, we instigate a regular daily meeting at 7.30 a.m. Every morning, the remaining Reception team file in. Young and old, facing their fears, plucky foot soldiers of the NHS.

We shut our doors to walk-in patients. In-person appointments are carefully managed so only a few people sit in the waiting room at any one time. Consultations take place in one of our three infection-controlled 'red rooms'. For those who can't travel but who need a doctor face to face, we follow careful protocols, which allow us to visit them in their homes.

*

The wind picks up my thin plastic apron and blows it up into my face. I push it down with gloved hands as I try to fit on my mask and visor. Although by now I've had a lot of practice managing my PPE, infection control is still tricky in the wind. It would be easier if I moved down the stairs and donned it in the tiny square foot of shelter immediately outside my patient's door. However, I sensed the urgency in the man's voice who spoke to me earlier on the phone. It's therefore pretty likely, I think, that he will fling open the door the second he knows I'm standing there. This will place us almost on top of each other, and I need to ensure I've got protection on first. A couple walking past me crosses over to the other side of the road to avoid the flailing plastic coverings I am wrestling with. These once-innocent items are now the icons of this deadly pandemic.

Fully donned, I descend the concrete steps. The curtain in the window to the left moves and the door opens just as I reach the bottom. Patrick is holding it open. His hair is slicked back in a 1950s rocker style. He wears a large bright blue suit jacket with padded shoulders and black winkle-picker shoes. His face is taut and grey with worry. He has been crying.

Lesley and Patrick have been together since they were fifteen years old. They were both from the St Mary's Park area of Limerick City in Ireland. They were born in almost identical pebble-dashed houses on almost identical streets barely 500 metres from each other. In the early 1970s, they moved to Brighton, a fun-loving, carefree couple in their mid-twenties. They found a little base- ment flat near the sea, surrounded by pubs and bars and artists. Patrick worked doing odd jobs for local builders and Lesley worked in a corner store. They collected little Irish trinkets to remind them of home, which slowly overtook the horizontal surfaces in their comfortable, dark flat.

In the fifty years of being here, Patrick hasn't lost his strong Irish accent – so much so it has been hard to understand him on the phone.

Lesley's case has been passed over to me by one of our GP col- leagues, Anna. She has been calling patients on her telephone list. She knows Patrick well already. A few years back, he nearly died of a pulmonary embolism – a blood clot in the lung. He walked around barely able to breathe for over a week before seeking any help. Patrick and Lesley didn't want to bother anyone. They carried on as if everything was fine, even when it clearly wasn't.

Given this history, Anna is very worried about the symptoms Patrick has described in Lesley. She has been vomiting for a few weeks and unable to keep much down. Over the last few days, she's started coughing and struggling to breathe. He doesn't know if she has a temperature; he doesn't think so. She had a bad night last night.

She had to sit in her chair all night, unable to breathe if she tried to lie down.

Anna has tried to get her seen in Brighton's new COVID HOT HUB, an assessment clinic that's been rapidly set up, but so far we've not been very successful in getting anyone treated there. They have strict regulations. The patient has to drive to the hub and remain in their car while being examined through the open door. A lot of our patients don't have cars or are feeling too unwell to use them. Neither Patrick nor Lesley knows how to drive.

Patrick ushers me into the house. The air is close and very warm. The curtains are drawn and the fire is on. Lesley is sitting on the sofa, a jaunty patchwork throw just visible behind her. Her eyes are fixed on a point in front of her, her shoulders moving up and down rapidly. She is concentrating hard on breathing. She turns her head slightly as I arrive next to her and tries to smile.

'T'would ya like a boiled egg?' Patrick asks me.

'Err, no, I'm okay, but thank you,' I reply.

I listen to Lesley's chest and put the sats probe on her finger.

Her heart rate is very high at 150 beats per minute, but her oxygen saturations are normal. She has fluid in the bottom of her lungs. I can hear the blood rushing over her mechanical heart valves. Her temperature is normal too, but she is very unwell. She could have contracted Covid, but she could also be in heart failure because her replacement valves might not be working as they should. She needs to go to hospital as soon as possible or she will almost certainly die.

I explain to them both that an ambulance will come and collect her. Lesley nods, and Patrick's face cracks as he stares down at the old Nokia phone in his hand.

'I can't work the phone, like, on my own,' he says. 'Lesley does that.'

It must be forty degrees in the flat. By now, my face is sweating under my mask. I can hardly breathe myself. I am dying to get outside into the cool fresh air. There is sweat running down inside my gloves. I pick up the couple's mobile phone, but it's dead. We find a charger and plug it in. That phone will be important in the coming weeks. Then I hurl myself out of the flat and sit on the lower step. I should take my gloves off first, but I can't wait – I pull my mask down and take off my visor, drawing the windy, sunlit air deep into my lungs along with a face-full of plastic apron. After double-bagging my unruly PPE and cleaning my equipment, I head back to the practice.

I call the hospital admissions number and ask to speak to the admitting consultant. I explain the situation and give Lesley's details, medication and past medical history. She is on an immunosuppressant drug for a rheumatological condition and multiple heart medications.

'Sounds like Covid,' says the medical consultant on the other end of the phone.

'Yes,' I reply. 'It could be, but it could be heart failure. She has a cardiac history.'

'Have you read the WHO guidance on Covid?' the consultant asks cheerily, and without criticism in her voice.

'Not all ninety-one pages of it,' I admit.

'Oh – you should, it's very helpful. Covid often has gastro symptoms. That's why there was such a run on toilet paper.'

I am not convinced by this assessment of the hysterical panic-buying of loo roll that dominated the UK's national news for a few weeks in the spring, but decide not to get diverted.

She continues: 'I'm afraid Lesley doesn't fit the criteria for ventilation, so there is really no reason to admit her. Her oxygen saturations are above ninety. She will have to stay at home. Call us back if her oxygen saturations drop.'

'She might have something else,' I reply. 'I think she could die if she stays at home with a heart rate that high.'

'Well, she might, but at the moment she does not fit the guidance for admission, sorry.'

She clicks the phone down.

I sit there for a while. This decision doesn't seem right. I also know there are eighty unused potential ITU beds standing in the hospital, ready and waiting for the expected rush of Covid victims. It feels to me as if 'Protect the NHS' – the slogan that's been plastered across all the pandemic press conferences given by government ministers and senior officials in recent weeks – may have gone a step too far. I pick up the phone again.

After several attempts, I manage to get through to a cardiology registrar called Tom who agrees to admit Lesley, bypassing the usual processes. Thank God for doctors like Tom. Lesley is taken to the Royal Sussex within hours.

I phone Patrick the next day. He hasn't slept. The ambulance took Lesley to hospital yesterday afternoon and he hasn't heard from her or the ward since.

'I just keep looking at her little cardigans hanging up and her things in the bathroom. We've not had a day apart in sixty years.'

I try to find which ward she is on by checking the names of the consultants ordering the blood tests, which I can see via our computer system. It looks like she is on the cardiology 'red' ward, for patients with suspected coronavirus as well as other health issues. So although there were no positive COVID-19 tests on her list of results, they obviously thought this was a possibility. I give Patrick the phone number and promise to call them and him the next morning, which is Saturday and might be quieter.

The next day, I log on to the results list under her name. There has been a flurry of activity overnight: CT scans and X-rays and bloods with various clinical indications including 'ventricular fibrillation – cardiac arrest'. She nearly died. Her heart was barely beating.

I call Patrick, but the phone is unavailable. I wonder if it has run out of battery again. I try again later that afternoon. His neighbour has helped him with his phone and he has spoken to the ward. His voice is quiet, and I'm not sure he is taking much in.

'I need to see her,' he repeats, over and over again. 'She will be so scared without me. I do all the talking, you see. Please can you help me?' I want to help but visiting rules are uncompromising at the moment. No relatives. Period. The risk of infection is too high. I promise to call again soon.

Day by day, we slowly track her course through the hospital. Cardiac ward, ITU, cardiac ward, back to ITU, cardiac ward again and then an elderly care ward. After three weeks, she is discharged home.

I call to see how she and Patrick are doing. Lesley has had a pacemaker fitted with a transmitter device, which needs to sit by the side of the bed. I imagine the terror on Patrick's face as he wrestles with the transmitter instructions. I imagine Lesley sitting on the sofa, her cardigan hanging off her diminished little frame, probably eating a boiled egg.

CHAPTER 14

Lockdowns

Terry Clark and his raging diabetes have been improving for quite a long time. It's taken lots of patience, and I know that our hard-won gains are fragile. He's still holding on by his fingernails. Now the pandemic has thrown a wrecking ball into many people's lives – and Terry is one of them.

The LGBT choir he attends has to close. All face-to-face contacts with our therapists are halted. There are no more acupuncture sessions with Ben. Terry begins to slip downwards, back into the Damp. One morning in June 2020, Emma, project manager of the Healing Arts Group, comes to see me, looking deeply distressed.

'Laura – I'm worried about Lizzy. Some of the cases she's been dealing with are really taking it out of her.'

I know Lizzy, who is one of our link workers. In normal times, she coordinates and supports patients as they access groups and resources. Like Emma, she gives her heart and soul to her job. During the pandemic, she has stepped up to the plate and helped to form the practice's Covid Support Group. The group works hard to stay in contact with the vulnerable and lonely, giving them attention and support. We've been in lockdown for three months, and I believe their work is saving lives.

'I think she's burning out,' Emma goes on. Her brow is furrowed. She massages her left palm absent-mindedly with her right thumb.

'She's working very long hours and spending a lot of time talking to extremely distressed people. I think it's really affecting her.'

'Who is she finding hardest to manage?' I ask.

'Definitely Terry Clark,' Emma told me. 'Things aren't good with him. She told me how difficult she's been finding it.'

'Right,' I said. 'I know Terry. Tell Lizzy I'll be calling him today.'

I have to try him several times. Eventually he picks up the phone.

'Hi, Terry, it's Laura, Dr Marshall-Andrews.'

There's a very long pause.

'Hello,' he eventually replies.

'Terry, I was just calling to see how you are coping with everything?'

His second pause is even longer.

'Not great.'

I wait for a while to see if he will elaborate, but nothing comes.

'What's been happening?' I try again to get him to speak.

'Well, I stopped taking all my meds for a bit. I didn't really see the point, y'know?'

'Yes, I can imagine. It's been really hard.'

'Lizzy really helps me. She calls me every Tuesday morning. I look forward to that. I think I'd end it if she didn't call.'

Already I can sense his depression seeping down the line, sapping my energy. I feel like giving up. I understand why Lizzy has been finding this so difficult.

'What has Lizzy been saying to you?' I ask him.

'She helped me with some food parcels, and – yeah. We just chat, really.'

'What are your blood sugars like?'

'They're bad.'

'How bad is bad?'

'Seventeen, eighteen. Sometimes twenty. Sometimes more. I dunno.'

A normal blood glucose level is between four and seven.

'Are you getting out at all, Terry?'

'No. I've not been out since – I dunno. Maybe March, or something.'

'You can go outside, you know. That's in the guidelines.'

'Yeah, Lizzy keeps saying. She's trying to get me to go on a walk or something – a photography walk.' He heaves a deep sigh, as though even the thought of doing this is exhausting.

'Maybe you should try it?'

'Yeah, maybe. We'll see.'

'Are you taking your medication again now?'

'Yeah.'

'Okay. I'll call you again in a couple of weeks, Terry.'

*

I go back to Emma and ask about how Lizzy is doing.

'When was the last time she took a break?' I enquire.

'I don't think she ever really stops,' Emma tells me. 'There are so many people suffering. All our online groups are full. We've been helping local food banks to distribute parcels, but the food banks can scarcely cope with demand. There've been people on the phones to us with nothing to eat.'

'What's happened to the local befriending service?'

'That's closed down. So has the counselling service.'

I try not to show Emma how bleak I feel as I listen.

'You guys are filling a big hole,' I say to her. 'Can we get any volunteers to help you take the calls? What about asking the Reception team?'

'Could we do that?'

'I'll certainly ask,' I tell her. 'If we can put support in, perhaps a few of Lizzy's most challenging cases can be taken off her for a while, to give her a break.'

As I walk home that day, I pass an engineer kneeling on the ground in front of an opened telecoms box. The multicoloured wires sprawl out as he works on their connections, like the inside of a robotic mind. They look to me like the complex neural connections of our captive community. I think of our Covid Support Group as a nerve centre of compassion, sending out its lifesaving data bytes of love and kindness. I only hope we're doing enough to keep the most vulnerable people in our community going.

*

A few weeks later, I speak to Emma again.

'We've just got back from the Deep Time group, Laura,' she tells me.

Deep Time walks are her brainchild, with the help of the National Park Trust. The group takes patients up to the Downs to follow the beautiful paths along the coast. The idea is that they can take photos, but participants are also encouraged to draw and talk as they walk along. The walks are reflective and mindful and, perhaps most importantly, they reinforce how easy it is to immerse yourself in nature – beauty really is just a bus ride away. People who take these walks often tell us how much better they feel – it's rare not to want to go again.

'A whole bunch of patients went up to Seven Sisters cliff, and walked a little way across the Downs. It was beautiful. Actually, Terry Clark came with us.'

'That's great.'

'It was. He did really well.'

'Say well done to Lizzy,' I told her. 'Terry appreciates everything she's doing. It may not always seem like it, but she really makes a difference.'

'Thanks. I'll tell her. But Laura – I don't know how much longer we can manage to keep going,' Emma says. 'I keep thinking, let's just pray we don't lock down again.'

'I'm praying,' I reply.

*

It's quite late one hot evening in July. I'm making my last few evening phone calls. The final call is to Patrick and Lesley. I wonder how they are doing after their traumatic early lockdown experience.

After a few rings, Patrick answers.

'Hi,' I say. 'How are things?'

'Oh, pretty good. Can't complain.'

I notice straight away that he sounds a bit worried.

'And how's Lesley?'

'Doing well now, doc. We are going for a walk every day. I think she's better than she has been for a long time.'

'Is something bothering you, Patrick?'

He hesitates. Then, 'Yes,' he says, 'I wanted to talk to ya, actually. It's that box t'ing that came with Lesley's heart t'ing. We never could get it to work, y'know. Does that matter?'

'Well, it would be good if it was connected. Just in case anything happens. Then the cardiology team can monitor her heart rate.'

'Oh, I see.' He sounds doubtful.

'Is there a phone number on it?' I ask.

'Well, yes, but ya know, it's like – no one ever answers.'

I hear a burst of laughter and the chinking of glasses. Across the road from the practice, customers at the local Greek restaurant are eating out of doors. The tables are socially distanced, but it's the sound of something like normality. It's easy to forget for a moment that there's still a very serious national problem.

'Yes,' I say. 'I know. Everyone's still under quite a lot of pressure with the pandemic. Maybe you could call the cardiology team?'

'Umm...' He sounds reluctant and uncertain of this plan.

'Are they pretty hard to get through to as well?'

'Yeah. I sort of gave up.'

'Look – don't worry. We'll try to get someone out to show you what to do.'

'Thank you. I need to go now, Dr Marshall-Andrews. We have to get the accordion out – for the clap.'

'For the Clap for Carers, you mean? I thought that was finished.'

'Oh yes, well, I know the NHS one has – but our street carried on. Simon has a drum set and there's a couple at number thirteen – we thought they were right odd but turns out they play the piano and he brings his electric whatsit out. Lesley does a bit o' singing. We have a few drinks, like... not too much, mind.' I get the feeling that he added the last bit when he remembered he was talking to his doctor.

'That sounds great, Patrick. I approve. Having some fun is good for you.'

'That's right,' he agrees enthusiastically. 'Otherwise, what's the point?'

'So Lesley's not had any more chest pain or breathlessness?'

'No, no – none at all. I'd better get going now, but thanks for calling those guys about the box. I get all in a muddle, you know?'

'No worries, Patrick. You have a good evening.'

'Thanks, doc. You too.'

He clicks off the receiver. I think of them getting together in the street, looking forward to the joy that gives them. I wonder what changes it makes in their bodies and their brains: floods of serotonin and maybe dopamine, perhaps growth factors being released, increasing neuroplasticity and lengthening cell life. Whatever it is, it's life-enhancing, and I'm certain that it's very, very good for their health. It's getting them through.

Impulsively, I reach for the phone, wondering if some friends of mine would like to seize this warm, golden evening and meet up on the beach.

*

So when autumn comes, and with it the next awful wave of the pandemic, life seems even harder. For a while the sun was shining and we wanted to believe that the problem was solved, or at least that the crisis was receding. It turns out that this was premature.

The ever-changing rules to deal with the virus have us all confused by now. Since July, parts of northern England have been back under pandemic restrictions. In Brighton, everyone's been trying to keep up, working out who can meet, and where, and what's allowed. In October, the whole country is divided into tiers, with differing restrictions dependent on the number of Covid infections. It's hard for some of our patients to follow these constantly changing regulations. Finally, early in November, comes national Lockdown Two.

Just after it's announced, I head down one of Brighton's backstreets towards Troy's flat. Once a difficult, regular and angry visitor to the practice, who spent his appointments railing and desperate, he has been transformed through a combination of acupuncture and table tennis. For several years now, he's been stable and relatively calm. But the pandemic has changed his health for the worse.

It's very cold now. I walk past narrow white houses in the eerie quiet. No other person moves apart from me, my rubber-soled shoes barely making a noise as I pad through this forgotten world. At the end of the road is the seafront, its grey shingle extending into the grey waveless ocean, which seems to flow seamlessly into the pale grey sky. It is as though a soft, suffocating blanket has been laid gently over the earth, stilling the human race to silence.

Troy has fallen and hurt his back. I spoke to him earlier on the phone and he sounded in terrible pain. He was unable to deliver a complete sentence without crying out. He's too terrified to go to A & E in the pandemic, so I've headed out to him. For Troy, as for too many others, the lockdowns have merged into a long experience of loneliness. He's only left his flat once in nine months. It's not the fear of Covid that deters him – more that he has been infected by a different type of virus. He is the victim of a fear that's proved far more damaging and life-limiting to many than the respiratory illness that has triggered it.

For so many who teetered on the edge of mental illness before the pandemic, this contagion of anxiety has pushed them to and then over the edge. Unable to continue the stabilising strategies they rely on – their gym, their football group, their pub quiz or their choir – they have retreated into the unsafe, unhappy recesses of the isolated mind.

Since the pandemic's first wave hit and the lockdown saw everything close, Troy's world has shrunk down to his tiny flat. Unfortunately, the flat is next to one of Brighton's largest homeless hostels. He is surrounded by crack dealers and chaos, and all the support we've tried to build for him has vanished. He's terribly vulnerable.

Eight weeks into the first lockdown, he'd popped onto my radar after my secretary forwarded an email to me from him. It was dark, abusive and desperate. I tried calling him but received no reply. Then, several days later, he sent a picture of himself attached to an email – and it was shocking. He'd lost a lot of weight. His skin was ashen and flaking. He had huge open wounds up his arms, which looked like unhealed burns. I knew what these were: the chemical burns of injecting or 'slamming' crystal meth.

I called him several times that day. He didn't pick up. Over the next week a pattern emerged. We received hate-filled, coercive and threatening emails in the small hours of the night – and then nothing. Sam goes round to his house but there is no reply. Troy seemed to be living a nocturnal life. And he is not alone, despite the lockdown rules: his emails described chem-sex parties at his flat. There were deeply disturbing undertones of violence. We informed the police, who carried out a welfare check. They were worried, but couldn't act on the unreliable assertions he was making.

It was painful to watch his catastrophic decline after so long and be powerless to help. Troy was slipping back into the struggling margins of society – and during lockdown, I suspected that those margins were getting more crowded every day.

As we move through lockdowns, politicians start to refer to the toll on the nation's mental health. Acknowledgement is something, but the words still feel to me like an aside – almost throw-away comments, a box that they are dutifully ticking. For us in general practice, the crisis is massive. Suddenly, almost everyone on my daily call list has mental health issues. We are inundated with calls from patients with histories of depression and anxiety that have now been reactivated and exacerbated by the pandemic.

Worryingly, there are also increasing numbers of new patients for whom this was their first descent into the darkness of mental illness. Sudden job loss, financial uncertainty, and the feeling of restriction and confinement bite into people's resilience. The pressures of home-schooling children and working online stretch tempers and exacerbate family rifts. For those for whom family is not a safe and happy refuge, but a place of danger, lockdown is disastrous: as a national poster campaign grimly points out, abusers very often work from home. But suddenly, there's no support that we can offer: along with routine hospital treatment, the already struggling mental health services have pretty much shut down.

One morning shortly after receiving the photo from Troy, the doorbell rang at work. I was on duty, waiting to see a small number of patients who needed face-to-face appointments. Charlotte put on her face mask and visor, sanitised her hands and opened the door. Troy was standing there, a blanket wrapped around his shoulders and trailing on the ground. His hair was dishevelled and matted. He looked filthy, a layer of grime darkening his skin, his finger nails broken and blackened.

Charlotte started to speak to him, but I jumped up to assist her.

'Hi, Troy.'

'Doctor, doctor – please help me. I can't go on like this. I need help. No one is helping me. I need to see a psychiatrist. I am so unwell.'

'Okay, come in.'

I ushered him into the empty nurses' room. In its bright, sterile environment, Troy looked even worse. And he smelt. Badly.

I called in our Polish nurse, Lara, who had been taking bloods in the next room. She brought in a pile of dressings and a flow of instructions and observations.

'Darlin', darlin', what is this? What have you been doing? Oh my God – look at your arms! That is terrible, what a mess!'

Between us, we disinfected each suppurating wound, removed debris and bits of cloth and dirt that were encrusted within them. Then we carefully wound clean white bandages over his brutalised skin. He swore at us but didn't move away. We worked steadily until all the damaged areas were covered. It felt good to be able to do something to help him. There wasn't a hope in hell that he could see a psychiatrist, not through the usual channels and with this sort of recent drug use. It's so much easier to deal with physical injuries. I found myself wishing I could pour a cleansing liquid over his brain, healing the festering wounds that were there.

'Now Troy – how else can I help you?'

'I need to see a psychiatrist. I am not well. I'm seeing things. I haven't slept for four days.' He must have known that we were trying our best to help him, but suddenly his old suspicious hostility flared up. 'I have rights, you know! I've paid my taxes!'

I'm far from sure that this last statement is true, but no matter. He was sweating and moving with a fine tremor. His pupils were dilated and he randomly jerked his head towards the door as if expecting someone. He definitely had the vestiges of some sort of amphetamine in him.

'I will refer you, Troy,' I said, 'but the waiting list is long. And you should know that they are a bit funny about seeing people while they are still using.'

'They're just scared. I'll sue the lot of them! They want me to go to CGL! Change, Grow, Live – what kind of fucking name is that for a drug service?'

In his state of total emergency, I couldn't help but feel he had a point.

'Change, Grow, Live can't look after me! They don't know a fucking thing about crystal meth! They only deal with heroin. Neglect, Ignore, Die is more like it.'

'Let's take it one step at a time,' I said in the calmest voice I could find. 'First, you need to sleep. Let me give you a medicine for sleep that will also help your paranoia. I'll refer you and we can take it from there. You'll need to come back in for your arms. Will you do that?'

The fight left him. Tears started rolling down his face.

'I'm sorry, I'm sorry. I'm just a mess.'

'I know Troy, I know. You have been here before, remember, but we were able to help you. Try to tell yourself that this won't last forever. You will get better again. The Table Tennis Club will re-open and we'll get you back there. I'm going to ask our "in house" psychiatrist to call you while we wait for the psychiatrist at Millview. She doesn't prescribe Western medication, though. She is a homeopath. I think she's brilliant. Will you talk to her?'

He closed his eyes. I waited, really hoping he was going to say yes. He'd accepted acupuncture already, reluctantly at first, and benefited from it.

'Okay,' he replied.

He got up, shakily. Lara made him a cup of tea and he took it into the waiting room. Maureen walked past and sat down briefly next to him. She asked about his table tennis, tilting her head to one side and gently touching his arm.

'Lockdown will be over soon, Troy,' she said encouragingly. 'Then we can all go back to normal.' I think she really believes this in the spring of 2020. I believe it myself – or I want to.

*

Standing here in the bitter autumn wind, that all seems a long time ago.

Troy lives in a converted house near the sea front. The houses are Georgian, with lovely long windows and little balconies. But the street has fallen on hard times. Most are council owned and used as halfway houses for people facing problems. The big homeless hostel, Phase One, sits halfway down and there are usually a few familiar faces hanging around the wide Regency steps that lead up to the door.

There are three buzzers on the wall outside Troy's building. None of them have numbers or names next to them. There is a brownish coating on all of them. The bottom one is falling off and has been sellotaped back to its base. This hasn't really worked and it hangs forward, gripping on for dear life, exposing a melee of thin wires at its back. I take out my phone and call Troy's number.

'Are you here?' he stutters.

'Yes. I am just outside – can you buzz me in?'

He makes deep groaning noises. I imagine him dragging himself over to the door. The buzzer goes and I push the door open and climb the stairs to the first floor. His door is ajar and I knock gently as I enter.

The door pretty much opens straight into a wall. There is a narrow corridor that heads off to the left. It's so narrow that I have to carry my doctor's bag in front of me to fit: whoever converted this old building into flats was trying to fit as many units into it as they possibly could with scant regard for convenience or comfort. At the end is a very small room. Troy is lying on the ground, wearing brownish trousers and an old T-shirt with the Nike tick and 'JUST DO IT' emblazoned across the front.

Daylight is blocked by a piece of material hung across the window. A plastic Christmas tree lies capsized in the corner. It's not Christmas for another five weeks, and I wonder if this is an early festive thought or whether the room has been stuck in a post-Christmas time vortex for the last eleven months. I think the latter: Troy is not the only one for whom 2020 has seemed like one unchanging, excruciating day.

I put my bag down and kneel next to him. He's in a lot of pain.

'What happened, Troy?' I ask.

'I just fell backwards from kneeling down. I was trying to fix the tap on the basin, but I fell onto a wooden box.'

We go through a basic neurological examination. He has good feeling in his feet and normal reflexes. There's power in his legs but moving them is painful. His arms are moving normally and he has no numbness over his pelvis or around his bottom. The pain in his back is between his shoulder blades. It's very tender on pressure. He really needs to go to A & E, but he point-blank refuses.

'I can't go there. I won't go there. Please, please don't make me.'

'Well, I can't make you, Troy, but it would be really good to image your back. I really think you should go. I can call an ambulance. They will be kind to you.'

'They know me,' he says flatly, 'and they won't be kind to me. They think I'm a drug addict.'

'Okay. Well – you don't have signs of damage to your spinal cord, which is good. It wasn't a violent injury, so that's reassuring too. But you're in a lot of pain. I can try to get you an X-ray at the Polyclinic. You can go straight there and straight back. There's no risk from the virus. I can send the request over and get you an ambulance.'

He agrees to this and I go back to the surgery to organise the X-ray and the ambulance.

Later that day comes a call from Troy.

'Did you get there?' I ask eagerly.

'I got there all right. It was fucking painful, though. The ambulance crew were great. But then they wouldn't do the X-ray. Said you shouldn't have sent me. What the fuck?'

'Oh Troy, I am so sorry. They should have done it. I checked the guidelines and they offer thoracic spine X-rays. Look – you will have to go to A & E, Troy. You can't stand up.'

'I'm not going,' he says shakily. 'I'll get Paul to come round and look after me.' He heard me draw breath to speak, and cut across me. 'I'm not going there! It's hell!'

'Okay. I'll refer you to the spinal clinic – you should be seen in five days. Don't move around too much and I'll call you every day.'

'Will they see me, though? Or will they turn me away too? I'm just not worth their while.'

'That's not the reason, Troy,' I say, just hoping he'll believe me. 'They don't think that at all. It's the pandemic. The services are so much more restricted than usual. They're scared of being overwhelmed.'

'That's just shit,' he replies, and I have to agree with him. The whole situation is just that.

I write an angry letter to the radiology department for turning him away. I don't get any response. In the end, Troy's urgent spinal referral takes four weeks to come through. He eventually makes it to an MRI scanner and gets home. It's another two weeks before we can track down the results. He has a fracture in one of his vertebrae, which is 'healing nicely with no cord impingement'. He is referred for physio, which may take some time. I ask Jess, who gave Troy some of his acupuncture sessions, to contact him again, to see if she can help with his discomfort.

Back at the practice, I tell Sam about what's been happening to Troy.

'The hospital is screwed,' Sam says. 'It's really not their fault. They were running on fumes before they shut down. Now they just don't have enough fuel in the tank to start up again.'

'Can you believe they turned him away at the Polyclinic?'

'Unfortunately – yes. I can believe it very easily. It's the same everywhere.'

I remind myself that we are luckier than most. We have the Robin Hood Health Foundation to back us up. That means there's help for our patients that they wouldn't find in many other places.

A few weeks later, when I telephone Troy, he sounds a little more upbeat when he answers.

'Hi, doc.'

'How's your back now?' I ask him.

'It's all right. Still a bit painful if I've been standing up for a while. Jess has been helping me again.'

'She's been good for you, hasn't she?'

There's a silence. Then he said simply: 'She got me off meth.'

'Does she still call you every week?'

'Yeah – every week for an hour.'

He paused.

'She said in Chinese medicine that I was a Snake!'

'They make odd diagnoses sometimes, don't they?' I said. 'How did that make you feel?'

'Well... ' he said. 'Well – I kinda get it. It makes sense. The way I would strike out at people. That was because I was scared.'

It does make sense, I thought. It really, really does.

'She gives me tablets,' Troy went on, 'but I think it's talking to her that really helps.'

'Are you still taking the olanzapine at night? The tablet I gave you.'

'Yeah, I'm still taking that one. When d'ya reckon I can stop?'

'Why don't we wait until you can get out a bit more and go back to table tennis and stuff before we worry about it?'

'Yeah, all right. Thanks, doc.'

'I'll call you again in a month, okay? But you can call me anytime if things get worse.'

'Yeah,' he said. 'Okay. And doc – just one more thing.'

'What's that, Troy?'

'When d'ya reckon this will all be over?'

We're constantly being asked this question. How long can the pandemic go on?

'I don't know Troy. I honestly don't know.'

He doesn't speak, but I can feel his silent dread.

'I think we will be freer in the spring,' I tell him. 'They're getting really close with the vaccines. That should help. I should think you'll be playing table tennis outside by Easter.'

He gives a long, exhausted, desperate sigh.

'Just keep getting up in the morning, Troy. Just keep getting up in the morning. Call me if you need anything.'

'Yeah,' he says, and clicks off the phone.

I put down the receiver too and reflect on our conversation.

He said, 'Thanks, doc.' He's calm. He's not swearing at me or making veiled threats. He's been injured, traumatised, but yet he's managing quite well. What's helping him to do this? Is it the shock of his back injury? Is it the tiny dose of olanzapine? Is it Jess's painstaking weekly calls and mentalisation therapy, helping him to make connections between his thoughts and his feelings, then link these to his behaviour? Or is it the sugar tablets infused by water (with a 'memory' of snake venom, as the homeopathic method describes it) dropped carefully onto them?

I feel sure that it is the mentalisation therapy. Jess's patience and her extraordinary ability to listen and help reframe events is a huge part of her successful treatments. I don't know about the sugar pills – but I know that there is power in intention. Jess believes the pills work, and that conviction of hers is transferred to some of those she treats. The belief that the patient and the clinician have in a treatment can have a significant effect on outcome. Harvard University now has a whole department of Mindset Medicine, studying the impact of this.

What's helping Troy, I think, is everything we've done – a combination of all of us working together. We have integrated these different systems, and together we have treated him as a whole person. We have made a difference.

Homeopathy is one of the more disputed alternative therapies. Personally, I think about it in terms of ethics. In medicine, we have four ethical pillars: Beneficence (do good), Non-maleficence (do no harm), Autonomy (value the independence of the patient) and Justice (ensure as much equity and fairness of care as possible). So in ethical terms, an ideal treatment is one that evidentially benefits patients, does no harm, is cheap and available to everyone. Not many of our medications or surgical procedures can boast this. But I'd say homeopathy comes pretty close.

CHAPTER 15

Hope

The lockdowns haven't been terrible for everyone, of course. I speak to those who have found positives in this strange situation. There are families who have enjoyed the time together, parents who've been around and got involved in a way that they couldn't when they commuted every day and worked long hours in distant offices. Now they aren't so sure they want to go back to the way it was before, rushing off first thing in the morning and returning home only after their children are in bed.

Some relationships have come under severe strain during the pandemic. But others have benefited. I have one patient who was miserable, angry and on the point of divorce when Lockdown One kicked in. With her and her husband both placed on furlough, I feared the worst for them. However, they thrived. Without the stress of long working hours, they spent more time together, went for walks and tended to the house and their children. They remembered the pleasure of each other's company and realised they had confused the distress caused by relentless pressure at work with frustration and animosity for their spouse. Now they had time, they saw that it was not each other they were struggling with – it was unsustainable work requirements.

Having space and time to think was the great gift of the furlough scheme for many. People went for walks and watched as spring changed the landscape. They'd always been too rushed and distracted before to notice. The skies above Brighton cleared as the air pollution fell away. Many patients commented on the crystal clearness of the sea. Just for a moment, we glimpsed the positive changes that could happen if we stopped burning fossil fuels and overheating our planet, stopped poisoning the land and the sea. One patient even commented to me: 'Perhaps we are the virus and COVID-19 is Earth's vaccine.'

We've certainly paid a high price to see all of this. But nature has a way of correcting imbalance, I guess.

*

For many people, though, it's just been tough.

The Burnells are a deeply good couple. They have committed their lives to bettering themselves and the world around them. Peter Burnell was a teacher and then a headmaster. He is fondly remembered by many of his staff and pupils who still contact him with missives of thanks and updates on their successes. He is kind and wise, with a slow and gentle scholarly demeanour that cannot be rushed.

Leila Burnell is all motherly love. She was born in Iran to a wealthy family there. In the days when they came into the surgery, she would bring me dates and dried berries sent from her family in Zarabad. I always enjoy seeing her; she is funny and interesting. She suffers from Obsessive-Compulsive Disorder and her hands are often raw and cracked from relentless washing and sanitising. She also suffers with Irritable Bowel Syndrome, which we manage with an array of different medications, fairly unsuccessfully to be honest. She still manages to keep her gentle sense of humour, but I know that her problems wear her down more than she lets on.

The most successful treatment she has found is our singing group. After several months of singing in our waiting room on Saturday mornings, she noticed that her IBS symptoms were lessening and she was not washing her hands and disinfecting the house so much. She persuaded Peter to join and together they became some of the most enthusiastic members of the group.

'He won't miss it – not for anything,' Leila tells me.

In 2015, aged 86, Peter had a massive heart attack. He had a quadruple bypass operation, then a post-operative infection, and spent four stormy weeks in hospital. Leila swore to me at the time that she was never going back into hospital, *not ever* again.

'Seriously, Laura, do you know the true meaning of bedlam? Well, that's what it's like up there.'

I looked up the word bedlam when she had left: 'a place, scene or state of uproar and confusion' is the dictionary definition. That did sound about right.

Peter had been very ill indeed. He was discharged with end-of-life medication and a DNACPR. He was not expected to live much longer. I went up to see him. He was lying in bed, pale and weakened by trauma and long periods of immobility. He barely spoke and Leila was worried as he was not eating or drinking much at all. Suspecting he might be approaching the end, I called in the district nurses and prepared for his continued decline.

But two weeks later, Leila rang me.

'He's singing!' she said.

For a moment, I thought this might be an Iranian way of saying he was dead.

'What do you mean?'

'He's singing! Some of the singing group came up to the house and sang by his bed and he joined in! It's a miracle.'

Several days later I called by their house on my way home. Peter was sitting up in bed and eating a crumpet. He looked like a completely different person. I couldn't believe it. Ever since I'd seen what singing

248

had done for Elizabeth's lung disease, I'd been convinced that it could help patients heal – but this really was incredible. So excited was Leila by the transformation that she hired a local opera singer to come and sing with Peter when the singing group was unavailable.

Was it just singing, or a natural bounce back after the traumas of hospital? Who knows. But within a few months, Peter was walking a few metres with a frame. A year after his big operation, he made it back to the Saturday singing group amid much celebration. Leonard Cohen's beautiful song 'Hallelujah' reverberated with an extra meaning around the practice that day.

Life went on for Peter and Leila. Despite their extreme frailty, they are devoted parents and grandparents, and in early 2020 they were looking forward to the birth of their first two great-grandchildren. It was looking like a wonderful year.

Then the pandemic hit and their lives capsized.

They are both on the extremely vulnerable list. I call them early on, in April 2020, to see how they're doing.

'We are okay, Laura,' confirms Leila. She sounds quite upbeat and chirpy. 'I have it all sorted. The virus takes three days to die. So we have a holding system for the post with Tupperware boxes in the hall. We leave any mail that comes in for at least that long. Then when I pick them up, I still use my plastic gloves. It's probably not strictly necessary, but it does make me feel better.'

'What about food?' I ask her.

'Oh – that's easy. I just ask the delivery man to leave everything in the old coal bin. It's quite cool in there. Then after three days, we fetch it indoors.'

I decide that they are pretty safe from Covid. Food poisoning, though, might be a hazard. But it's not all that likely, so I don't say anything. I don't want to scare her, and everything sounds complicated enough as it is.

Then I don't hear anything from the Burnells for months and months. I know that the practice's Covid Support Group is contacting them weekly. The singing group has moved online, which is wonderful for some of its members, but the Burnells don't have those kind of computer skills.

One Monday morning in January 2021, I pick up a panicked call from Leila.

'Oh Laura, oh Laura, it's Peter! We had the paramedics out over the weekend. He is so poorly. They did a test and we heard today, he's got Covid. How could he have got Covid? I did everything I could. Will he die?' She is sobbing hard and her voice is shrill between gulps of air. 'How can he have Covid, Laura – how?'

'I don't know, Leila. Have you been out at all?'

'No, no, we haven't! No since the first of March last year. We haven't seen our children or grandchildren for ten months. We haven't seen our great-grandchildren at all, *ever*. Oh – how could this happen? He is so ill.'

'What did the paramedics say?'

'They said he wasn't sick enough to go to hospital – but maybe they just need the beds!' She bursts into uncontrollable crying again.

I wait for her to calm down, and while I do, I quickly find her records on my screen.

'I can see the paramedic report now, Leila. It looks like his oxygen saturations were really good when they saw him. He was breathing quickly but he was okay. Leila, remember – most people survive this.'

'Even if they are ninety-two years old with a serious heart condition?'

'Yes, most people like him will still survive a Covid infection. He is at greater risk of problems, certainly, and we need to monitor him carefully. But he has a good chance of being okay. Have you got a pulse oximeter?'

'Yes – my son bought us one from Amazon last year.'

'Great. And a blood-pressure monitor?'

'Yes.'

'Okay. So I will phone you every day and we can monitor him at home. If his saturation drops below 92 per cent, you call me here. If it drops below 90 per cent, you call 999, okay? We'll try our best to keep him out of bedlam.'

She sniffs. 'Thank you, Laura.'

I put the phone down and say a prayer for them both.

Over the next ten days, Peter's oxygen saturations teeter around the 92–93-per-cent mark. He spends most of his time in bed. On day ten I make my afternoon call to Leila.

'Hi, Leila, it's Dr Laura.'

'Hi, Laura. Well – today is a big day. Peter's up! He had a shower and he is sitting in his chair with a blanket over his knees. He had some soup and he asked for more.'

I almost burst into tears with relief.

'What are his oxygen saturations?' I ask her.

'They are 94 per cent now but they were 96 per cent this morning – the best ever. Oh Laura, I think he's going to be okay. I really do. I can't believe I haven't got it too. I really thought we were both going to die.'

'I understand, Leila. It must have been terrible.'

'I wasn't even that worried about me dying, you know?' she tells me. 'All I could think was – at least I won't have to learn how to use a computer now.'

'Oh my goodness,' I say.

We agree to move to twice-weekly phone calls and slowly, slowly Peter improves. They are still locked in a prison of fear within their house, but I am hopeful they will be able to venture outside at least once or twice a week. Perhaps they could see their family at a distance in a park or on the beach, I suggest to Leila. But she's adamant. She won't take any risks at all after everything she's been through.

'We'll wait for the vaccine,' she says. 'Will you call us when it's our turn?'

'Yes,' I reply. 'It's coming. It won't be long now.'

*

I am walking along the seafront. It's still dark but the sun is just beginning to appear above the horizon. It feels like it's been cold and raining for months. The damp chill seeps into your core after a while. This winter has seemed so very long. Now, in mid-February, it feels like the country is on its knees, desperately crawling towards that glimmer of hope that still seems just out of our reach. A COVID-19 vaccine, and spring.

I pull my thick scarf closer around my face as the early-morning air bites at my exposed skin. I'm on my way to the vaccination centre. We have to get there thirty minutes before any patients arrive, to start drawing up the Pfizer vaccine. It's hard to think of a more challenging process.

This vaccine itself needs to be stored at -70 degrees. Once out of those conditions, it can stay active for five days at normal fridge temperatures. Once it's taken out of the fridge, at normal room temperature, it has a six-hour life span. Like some rare butterfly, this long-incubated substance has a brief but glorious existence.

So GP practices across our area have been taking part in long online planning meetings, working out how to distribute it. The challenge is to ensure that the largest possible number can benefit, and that none of it is wasted. But the suppliers can't be sure when they will deliver the vaccine, or exactly how much they will deliver. Even when they can tell us how many vials will be arriving, we can't be 100-per-cent certain how many vaccine doses we will get from each one. It could be four or five, or even six doses, if the vaccinator is careful. For this is no normal vaccine. The liquid cannot be disturbed or the delicate lipid capsule that transports it will be disrupted and the vaccine rendered useless.

The outcome of our planning is that thousands of patients are on standby, waiting for the call so we can race to get the precious fluid into their arms. We have teamed up with nine other practices and I am working out of the biggest practice's premises. They have a large car park – and spare rooms too, I notice with some envy.

I arrive at 7.30 a.m. The vaccination room, although barely warmer than the air outside, is well lit and friendly. There is bunting hanging on the walls and the general feel of a church fete. I change into my scrubs and present myself to the team leader, a tall GP called Anna.

'Ah yes, Laura – you are working with Helen, over in the corner there,' she directs me. I know Helen, who works in a neighbouring practice. I've always found her light-hearted and fun. She is in her early thirties with dark, shiny hair. This morning I notice that she's wearing Sweaty Betty thermals underneath her scrubs. I feel another pang of envy. She's clearly worked in this chilly room before.

'Hi, Laura, is this your first time?' she asks me brightly.

'Yes,' I reply. 'Frankly, I'm terrified!'

'You'll get the hang of it. You just have to be very, very slow with your movements, especially when making up the vaccines. I'll run you through it.'

She moves over to the table. There's a box of vials sitting there, nestling in their dark foam holders like expensive jewellery. There are slender syringes and blue needles laid out carefully by the side. The vaccine box sits on a card, which reads: 7.00–13.00.

'That's our time frame for those vials,' Helen explains. 'Do you want to start drawing up or injecting? It's quite intense drawing them up – you have to be so careful and slow. It's not great on your back either. And your eyes go a bit funny after a while. We'll need to switch over after a few hours.'

I opt for drawing up and settle into position. I am determined to get six injections out of every vial. If you manage this, you shout 'six'. Then the planning team can increase the appointment slots and call in more patients. I take out the first vial and move it carefully onto a blue plastic tray. I take a deep breath and then slowly, so slowly, inject 1.6ml of water into the vial. My arms shake slightly with the effort. The vial must then be inverted ten times to mix the liquids, but again this must be a smooth, slow movement, backwards and forwards, no shaking or sudden jerks. I put the vial slowly down on the tray and move back to shake my arms out. I'm feeling tense. Now for the drawing up. I take my first slim syringe, attach the blue needle and with infinitesimal downward movements of the plunger, draw the milky fluid, drop by precious drop, into the body of the syringe.

I manage to get six doses lined up on the tray. I shout: 'I have six!' This feels like a cross between bomb disposal and a TV game show.

After a couple of hours, just when I think I've gone permanently cross-eyed and can no longer feel my legs, Helen suggests that we switch places. I take up my new position by the prepared syringes. There are four tables of doctors and nurses drawing up and injecting. We are the closest to the door. I call the first patient over and sit him down. He pulls up his sleeve and we run through the check list. The last question, 'Is there any chance you could be pregnant?' makes him laugh. He is eighty.

After about an hour and much joviality, I see Peter and Leila Burnell waiting at the door. I call them over to my vaccination table. They are both wearing blue plastic gloves and visors over their masks. Leila is pushing Peter in a wheelchair.

'Oh Laura – we're so glad we got you,' Leila says. 'Isn't this marvellous? Everyone has been so kind. I can't believe it. I can't believe it's really happening.'

She takes a seat on one of the plastic chairs. I inject them both with my vials of liquid hope.

Leila stands up.

'Thank you, Laura, thank you. We will try to get outdoors soon.' Tears well up in her eyes and she pats Peter on his shoulder. 'We'll see the kids soon, love.'

He shuts his eyes tight and reaches up to hold onto her hand. He nods his head. He can't speak. Neither can I.

The rest of the morning goes quickly and soon I'm saying goodbye to Helen and packing up. Jacqui arrives to take over. There's a long way to go yet – but maybe, just maybe, we're getting there.

I decide to walk back along the sea front. There are a few walkers and cyclists out. Sea swimmers take the plunge off Brighton beach, even in the cold months of the year. I can see several sitting there now, their large dry robes fanning out around them. The sun hovers behind a cloud.

As I walk along the side of the Level, Brighton's central green space, I notice that the daffodils are out. Hundreds of them line the long pathway. I think of them pushing their way up through the cold, dark soil to stand triumphantly in the sun. They are nature's perfect heralds of change. I feel my jaw soften and my shoulders relax. For a moment, I let a wash of hope and joy flood over me, pushing back the struggle and the pain.

It's okay. Spring is here.

Epilogue

It's just so much cheaper to help people stay well than to cure illness.

A recent study showed that every one pound spent on arts in health saved the NHS eleven pounds. This is money worth spending, because – in a crude, economically driven sense – the last thing you want is for people to be seriously ill.

To quote one of my favourite sayings, which was coined by Professor Francis Omaswa: 'Health is made in communities, hospital is for repairs'. GPs and primary care practices are perfectly situated within our communities to help create and promote good health, as well as to sift out the symptoms and signs of more serious active disease that requires hospital 'repair'. This is what we should be investing in.

I've learned from my patients that approaching every situation with the view that 'the doctor knows best' can mean closing off opportunities to listen and learn. Experience has taught me that good medicine – in the very broadest and most generous sense of 'good' – is what works. It works for patients and their families, and the wider communities of which they are a part. It's the only way to bring about the changes we need. I believe that the practice itself has become a living manifesto for that change. I'm deeply proud of this.

'Resilience' is a buzzword right now. There's so much talk about it that cynicism has started to creep in. Perhaps it's just the government's way of getting us to do more for less, a cunning ploy to extend our capability.

For me, real resilience has always come in the form of love and humour. It is about caring deeply for your patients – but not so much that it breaks you. It is about giving almost everything you have, but not everything. It's about knowing you have been true to your values and beliefs.

I have always been proud that the motto of the Royal College of General Practitioners is *cum scientia caritas*. This translates as 'science with love'. I hope we can help to swing the pendulum back towards recognising the value of kindness, and to reach beyond the textbook or the protocols.

When the ex-Chief Executive of the NHS, Lord Nigel Crisp, came to visit the practice, he and I were lamenting the difficulty in changing the current culture of the wider NHS. He looked at me and said: 'Change happens in the heads of the healthcare professionals.' I have always remembered that.

There is nothing stopping us from making the changes that are needed. Only ourselves. I think we want to do it. I also know we have to, for all our sakes.

Acknowledgements

Thank you to all the patients who kindly agreed to have their stories represented in this book, and to those who, over the years, have taught me so much about humanity.

Thank you to Hannah Vincent for her wisdom and edits in the very early days of writing this.

Thank you to Liz Sheppard (who I think is some kind of genius) who managed to help turn a motley collection of stories into a cohesive narrative.

Thank you to Claire Paterson Conrad for believing that that motley collection of stories could be something more, and to Kate Fox for guiding and inspiring the process.

Thank you to Abi Le Marquand-Brown, for the gigantic task of getting the book through the legal reading, and to Arthur Heard for his advice.

Thank you to Gabriel Weston for introducing me to Claire.

Thank you to the team at BHWC who have been like a family to me and whose humour and kindness have lifted the hardest moments, in particular to Gary, who has always been there for me.

Thank you to Dr Sarah Andersen for her blue sky thinking.

Thank you to Rich Des Veoux for all the commas and poesy.

Thank you to Tara for patiently listening to all these stories over the years.

Thank you to my parents for their enduring support and belief in me: to Mum for telling me all the bits that were unreadable as well as all the bits she liked, and to Dad for his story telling, which has coloured my life. I love you.

ONE PLACE. MANY STORIES

Bold, innovative and
empowering publishing.

FOLLOW US ON:

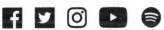

@HQStories